FOR THE
HURT
—— OF MY ——
PEOPLE

ORIGINAL CONSERVATISM

& BETTER, SIMPLER HEALTHCARE

JOSEPH Q. JARVIS, MD, MSPH

CONTENTS

Acknowledgments   vii
Introduction   ix

1. Health Care: The Gift We Give Ourselves   1
2. Avarice versus Altruism   7
3. State-Based Health Reform: What Conservatives
   Believe   20
4. Running through the Political Icebox   35
5. Health Care: The Sentinel Domestic Issue of
   Our Time   46
6. Metaphor and Healing   51
7. The Metaphorical Physician   66
8. The How of Progress and Conservative Health
   Reform   78
9. Harris Wofford, Force, and Harshness   85
10. Downstream Danger   97
11. The Bell Tolls for Every American   108
12. Biblical Wisdom and Original American
    Conservatism   130
13. Maximum Effort   141

What You Can Do   155
Notes   161
About the Author   165
Also by Joseph Q. Jarvis, MD, MSPH   167

*This book is dedicated to Hillary Jarvis and Margaret Jarvis,
my intrepid hiking companions, with love, from their father.*

EBook ISBN: 978-1-958085-00-4

Trade Paperback ISBN: 978-1-958085-01-1

Hardcover ISBN: 978-1-958085-02-8

Cover design by Suzanna Marie Collet

Cover artwork image, "Jeremiah, as depicted by Michelangelo from the Sistine Chapel ceiling." The Yorck Project (2002), public domain.

Interior print and eBook design and layout by Kailey Urbaniak

Production services facilitated by The Book Break

Scriptures taken from New Revised Standard Version Bible, copyright © 1989 National Council of the Churches of Christ in the United States of America. Used by permission. All rights reserved worldwide.

Published by Principle Print & Media

Principle Print & Media EBook Edition 2022

Principle Print & Media Trade Paperback Edition 2022

Printed in the USA

ACKNOWLEDGMENTS

I have devoted thousands of hours of volunteer time to the cause of changing how we Americans do health care business over the past three decades because I believe what Jesus of Nazareth taught His followers two thousand years ago, that it is my duty to see to the needs of the sick. Over these many years, as I have become persuaded that the United States of America is failing to care for the sick and injured, I acknowledge that I derive energy and commitment to the cause of reforming American health care delivery from the words and example of the Son of Man, who was Himself a Healer. To the extent that I succeed in this effort, all credit is due to Him.

I have been blessed again by the developmental editing skills of Kathy Jenkins and the copy editing capabilities of Michele Preisendorf. Melissa Dalton Martinez and her team help me make publishing decisions and make my public relations possible. Many thanks to these publishing professionals for the care and competence they have woven into this book.

My wife, Annette W. Jarvis, has become my publishing partner; together we have formed and own Principle Print and Media LLC. She makes it possible for me to carry on my advocacy work in health system reform, including writing this book.

A section of this book had its origins during my years in medical training at the University of Utah School of Medicine, while I was mentored by both Dr. Dona L. Harris and Dr.

Charles Hughes, both now passed on. I am grateful for what these two eminent scholars taught me and dedicate this book to their memory.

INTRODUCTION

America's healthcare system is an expensive mess. If you've had much to do with it, you know exactly what I'm talking about.

Everyone agrees on that. What we *can't* seem to agree on is how to fix it.

But the solution is really quite simple. We need better, simpler, and therefore cheaper care guaranteed for everyone without cost at the point of medical service. Health care should be delivered cooperatively across regions, with the patients' interest foremost, but instead we have competing corporate, for-profit interests that would rather make a sale than really take care of patients.

But wait—wouldn't health care for everyone be socialism? How can *that* be good?

No. It isn't socialism.

Let me explain the difference.

In a cooperative healthcare system, the taxes already paid by all citizens finance health care. No one has to get his or her own health insurance. No one has to pay out-of-pocket premiums, deductibles, copayments, or coinsurance for healthcare programs to get medically necessary care. No or only minimal out-of-pocket costs are incurred. No one has to sign up for health insurance. Babies are automatically enrolled at birth, and no one is ever disenrolled. Everyone is included in publicly financed and arranged healthcare delivery ideally run by each state instead of the federal government, though federal health care for all would certainly be better than the expensive, wasteful healthcare delivery currently used in the United States.

Publicly financed and privately delivered care for everyone isn't some sort of wild-eyed, radical idea. It's working very well in a number of first-world countries where taxes are enough to pay for all medically necessary services. And here's the amazing part: the other first-world countries tax themselves less for health care than we in the United States do.

So, how is that different from "socialized" medicine? In socialized medicine—which isn't used in most first-world countries—the government owns and operates all hospitals, hospices, nursing homes, rehab centers, clinics, dialysis centers, and other healthcare facilities. It also employs all the doctors, nurses, and other health professionals.

No one has ever seriously proposed socialized medicine for the United States. Senator Bernie Sanders proposed a system he calls "Medicare for All." Here's what he means by that: as is done in Canada, public funding would pay for private healthcare delivery. But unlike what is done in Canada, Sanders proposed a national payer for health care; in Canada, the federal government supports the various provincial governments, which then pay for privately delivered healthcare services. Could that work in the United States? Absolutely. In fact, a system of state-based public payers for private healthcare delivery already appears to have substantial support across the country and would therefore be more politically feasible in the United States than a national payer, such as Medicare for All.

And here's the important thing to understand: Americans

already pay enough taxes to finance medically necessary care *for every resident in our country without any out-of-pocket costs.* In order for this to work, though, the health-financing system must be simpler and the care better.

I'd like to show you exactly what I'm talking about with the tragic story of what happened to my friend. In order to protect her privacy, I have changed her name and some of the specific details of her life. But the rest of the story is true and provides an accurate depiction of the suffering and dilemmas she experienced through American healthcare malfeasance.

Ten years ago, Jenna Jones was a married thirty-year-old with two daughters. Her husband had a career in construction that provided enough income to house and feed his family. He also had health insurance through his employer. Sounds great, right? Not so fast. Let's take a closer look at the financial details of that employee "benefit."

The employer-provided health-insurance policy, in addition to costing the employer so much that wages at that business had been held down for years, also had many and various out-of-pocket expenses for Jenna's husband, such as premiums (beyond what his employer paid), copayments, deductibles, and coinsurance. In addition to all this out-of-pocket expense for his family's potential current healthcare needs, he—as do we all—paid remarkably high taxes for publicly funded healthcare programs, including federal taxes to support Medicare, Medicaid, Indian Health Service, Tri-Care, CHIP, VA Health Care, and an acronym soup of other federal healthcare programs. It didn't stop there—for him or for any of us: he also paid state and local taxes to support the state portion of the Medicaid and CHIP programs and the healthcare benefits for public employees, including elected leaders, teachers, municipal and other public employees, sewer-district employees, and other state and local healthcare programs. Taken together, more than two-thirds and maybe as much as three-fourths of the $4 trillion per year currently spent on healthcare programs comes from taxes. Jenna and her husband paid their share of that and *still* had to pay for their own health insurance plus significant out-of-pocket costs.

Jenna also worked. She was an entrepreneur with various business interests, including renting motor homes, marketing books, and selling fitness programs to senior citizens. Because she was "self-employed," she had no job-related health benefits; she was covered by her husband's health insurance.

During her late twenties, she had two normal pregnancies but gained significant amounts of weight each time. She tried but was unable to lose the weight. Her husband made the situation worse by telling her he was no longer interested in her because she was too fat.

The emotional fallout was significant, but there were also physiological issues. As her body mass index (BMI) ballooned into obesity, she began experiencing difficulty sleeping. Her physician told her she had sleep apnea due to being overweight. He prescribed a CPAP (continuous positive airway pressure) machine, which her health insurance partially funded. Her doctor said that if she lost weight, her sleep apnea might improve and she might not need CPAP.

Jenna looked into nutritional and fitness counseling, but the health insurer did not cover these services. Her husband decided not to pay for them out of pocket. Jenna began to feel depressed, but mental health services were also not a covered benefit, so she couldn't seek help for her depression.

When it appeared that her husband might leave the marriage, Jenna took drastic action. She asked her physician for a referral to a bariatric center. There, she received the testing and other services needed to document that she was a candidate for gastric-sleeve surgery. Though the health insurer paid for the bariatric clinic evaluation, it denied payment for the surgery. Once the bariatric clinic discovered she had no payment source for surgery, they dropped her.

But Jenna did not give up. She had been told she should have gastric-sleeve surgery—a surgery that reduces the size of the stomach, forcing the patient to eat less and therefore lose weight—so she looked for an alternative clinic to provide her with the surgery at a lower price. She found one such clinic in Tijuana, Mexico, that offered the surgery for $2,000—one-tenth of the cost in the United States. Her husband, hoping to have a slim marriage partner again, agreed to pay out of pocket for the surgery. Jenna drove herself to Mexico and checked herself into the clinic.

The surgery, which is not minor in even the best situation, was an agony. Conditions in the hospital were not sterile. The recovery area was understaffed, the food substandard. She spoke no Spanish, so she couldn't understand what was happening. She was nauseated and vomited for several days after the surgery. There were drains coming out of her rather large surgical wound, her dressings were changed only intermittently, and she was in constant pain and couldn't rest.

Jenna was discharged before she felt at all well, and she had to drive herself back to Utah. There, she had to find a physician to provide her with postoperative care, including removal of the drains. The insurance refused to cover the cost of this care.

Since her surgery ten years ago, Jenna has never felt entirely well. She did lose weight—more than a hundred pounds—and her sleep apnea improved to where she no longer needed CPAP. But she continued to experience intermittent nausea and vomiting. Her surgical wound healed unevenly, leaving a large, unsightly scar on her abdomen.

Jenna's husband became sexually interested in her again for a time, and she became pregnant. This pregnancy, however, was complicated by frequent and severe nausea, vomiting, and placenta previa, where the placenta covered her cervix, putting Jenna at risk for rupture and life-threatening bleeding.

During Jenna's pregnancy, she was on bed rest for months

and unable to maintain adequate nutrition and hydration, which threatened the fetus. She began feeling depressed again. Whenever she tried to eat while lying in bed, she experienced heartburn. Fortunately, she delivered a healthy baby boy via C-section.

After the pregnancy, she continued to be depressed. And though she had fewer episodes of nausea and vomiting, the heartburn continued. She managed to keep most of the excess weight off, but her husband lost interest in her anyway. Two years after her son's birth, she separated from her husband.

Jenna supported herself by engaging full-time in travel marketing while also being a full-time, single mother. Her children stayed with their father only every other weekend. Her children had health insurance through their father, but there was no way Jenna could afford health benefits, so she had no financial support when she needed care. She developed asthma but could not seek treatment. She experienced increasing heartburn and reflux but simply purchased more Tums. She developed numbness and pain in her hands and could not afford to have it medically evaluated.

Before her son turned four, Jenna met and married her current husband, Fred. He worked at a software company and was able to include her on his health insurance. While there were still out-of-pocket payments to be made, she sought care for her various symptoms. But that didn't go well.

One physician told Jenna she needed carpal-tunnel surgery for the pain and numbness in her hand. She underwent the surgery but experienced no relief. She sought an additional evaluation elsewhere and was advised that her hand symptoms might be due to problems in her neck. This doctor advised an imaging study of Jenna's cervical spine, but her husband's health insurance denied the request, maintaining it was not necessary. Due to poor communication between the insurer and the doctor's office, the imaging study was conducted anyway; it documented several collapsed discs in the cervical spine with nerve impingement, clearly explaining the pain and numbness in her hand. None-theless, the health-insurance company insisted that the imaging study was not medically necessary and refused payment, which then fell to Jenna and Fred. This imaging study totaled $8,000.

During the most recent year, Jenna's heartburn increased. Tums no longer relieved the recurring pain in her chest. She had constant reflux even after eating minimal amounts of food. At night, she experienced coughing and choking when-ever she reclined. Her primary care physician prescribed acid-reducing medications, but even these did not help. She was referred to a gastroenterologist. After conducting a scope study of her stomach and esophagus, he told her that her esophagus was ulcerated and scarred. He diagnosed her with a hiatal hernia and referred her to a surgeon.

The surgeon Jenna consulted verified the diagnosis but said hiatal-hernia-repair surgery was not possible for Jenna because of her previous gastric-sleeve surgery. There simply was not enough of her stomach left to repair the hernia. He referred her to another surgeon experienced in repairing the substandard gastric-sleeve operations commonly conducted in Mexico.

The new surgeon was part of a bariatric service, one that specialized in weight-loss surgery. She proposed to Jenna that the only approach to helping her with her constant reflux and esophageal scarring was a gastric bypass, essentially connecting the esophagus to the small intestine. This surgery meant Jenna would permanently be able to consume only very small amounts of food and drink at a time. And she would also need to be selec-tive in her food choices since the small intestine could not tolerate some foods. Nonetheless, Jenna felt she needed the surgery. She was often dehydrated because she could not drink enough water without coughing and choking, and she was losing weight because she could not maintain adequate caloric intake.

Jenna tried to schedule the surgery, but her husband's health insurance denied the preapproval for payment, stating that she did not meet the criteria for a bariatric procedure. The surgeon submitted documentation that the surgery was necessary not because Jenna needed or sought weight loss but because her esophagus required protection from reflux and the consequent erosion and scarring from the acidic nature of her stomach's contents. The health-insurance company failed to respond to this additional information.

Jenna and her husband hoped to get the surgery done before the end of the year because they had already met the large deductible required by their insurance package. But the fight to gain insurance approval for the procedure was pushing the surgery into the new year, when she would have a large deductible to pay, along with other out-of-pocket costs.

And that's not all. *After* the open-enrollment period, the insurance company announced that their provider network was changing in the new year and Jenna's surgeon would no longer be an in-network provider.

Jenna and her husband had no other choice than to begin planning to pay for the surgery themselves, a cost of $40,000. Similar surgeries elsewhere in the developed world cost much less than half this amount.

Astonishingly, Jenna's problems with healthcare delivery are all too common in the United States. In any other first-world country, virtually everything about this story would have been different. For instance, had there been a public payer for all medically necessary privately delivered health care when Jenna first started experiencing weight gain, she could have received help with counseling, nutrition, and fitness before ever becoming morbidly obese and suffering from sleep apnea. Consider how perverse Jenna's situation was: insurance wouldn't pay to help her manage weight gain, but it did pay for a CPAP machine made necessary because of her obesity. Jenna would also have had assistance for her mental health issues, including those caused by an uncaring, neglectful, and abusive husband.

The bottom line? Had Jenna lived in a country with better, simpler, and therefore cheaper care, she probably would not have needed weight-loss surgery at all. She wouldn't have been forced to find cheaper, substandard surgery in Mexico, and she would not have ended up with esophageal ulcers, a truly debilitating and life-threatening condition that required a very invasive surgery to save her from gradual starvation and dehydration.

There were other problems too. For an entire decade, Jenna was plagued by the difficulties of claim denial, out-of-pocket costs, and unilateral changes in provider networks. In countries with better, simpler, cheaper systems of care, patients don't suddenly find themselves "out of network," surprised by bills, struggling to meet deductibles, or, having met the annual deductible, struggling to get a surgery done before the new year and its incurring cost of a renewed deductible payment. In first-world countries with better care, more simply financed patients are not denied payment by insurance companies for medically necessary care.

The entire American system is built on a flimsy foundation: tying health benefits to work itself is a massive problem. People feel compelled to stay in unproductive, unfulfilling jobs in order to keep their health-insurance benefits when they would thrive and better promote our common economy if allowed to be entrepreneurial or take other career risks. Some people, like Jenna, stay too long in harmful marriages, in part because their spouse has the health insurance, which they would lose if the marriage ended. These problems never occur in countries with public financing for privately delivered health care arranged for all.

If we want to fix our healthcare woes—calamities like the ones suffered by Jenna and countless other Americans faced with navigating a devastatingly ailing healthcare system—we must jettison our market bias and adopt a different model of health-care delivery in which cooperation and the needs of patients come first. We need to drop the pretense of markets in health care. We need to abandon business as usual in American health care, which is focused on nothing more than maximal profits.

We can either have the most profitable healthcare system in the world, or we can have better, simpler, cheaper care oriented to the needs of the patients. We cannot have both. We can't optimally help Americans suffering illness or injury if patients are not given priority over profits.

In the pages that follow, I'll show you how that can be done— and I'll start with a harrowing experience I had in the rugged mountains near my Utah home.

1
HEALTH CARE: THE GIFT WE GIVE OURSELVES

The helicopter circled within the steep canyon conclave, searching for someplace to stop, hold steady, and take on passengers. The rescuers could see where we were among the pines on the canyon sidewall in the fading sunlight of a June evening in Utah because my future son-in-law, Forrest Strech, had had the foresight to bring a flashlight on what became a twenty-five-mile trek.

We had started the day by parking my car at the gate to City Creek Canyon, just north of downtown Salt Lake City. Above the gate stretches five and a half miles of paved road, ending at a pavilioned picnic ground in the pines. Above the pavilions, a good trail continues more than five miles up into the Wasatch Front mountain range where Davis, Salt Lake, and Morgan counties converge. I had planned to lead my small group of hikers—including Forrest and his then girlfriend, my daughter Margaret, and her sister, my eldest daughter Hillary—triumphantly down City Creek Canyon long before dusk and drive home in my waiting Jeep Rubicon. We should never have needed a flashlight.

After leaving the Jeep at the mouth of City Creek Canyon, my small hiking group rode in Margaret's Subaru Impreza to the crest of East Canyon, a pass along the Mormon Pioneer Trail where Brigham Young caught his first glimpse of the Salt Lake Valley in 1847. We parked the Subaru on the shoulder of Big Mountain and began hiking along its west face on the Great Western Trail toward upper City Creek Canyon. It was a beautiful late-spring day high in the mountains, blue skies with bright, white piles of cumulus clouds spreading out above us.

Snowbanks were still melting along the trail, and as we skirted them, we enjoyed panoramic vistas along the east side of the Wasatch Front. By midmorning, we found a sign declaring that we were in the upper reaches of City Creek Canyon and warning us that it was a protected watershed.

Despite being in the upper reaches of the canyon, exactly where we needed to be, inexplicably, I yearned for a more challenging trail. In my nonsensical pursuit, I led the group mistakenly around to the north side of Grandview Mountain, which forms the northeastern rim of the canyon. As a result, instead of dropping down into City Creek Canyon, we descended into a smaller canyon to its north. There, we spent the afternoon fruitlessly searching for the good trail I had expected to find had we been in City Creek Canyon.

We had plenty of water and nourishment, but as the afternoon grew later and I—a generation older than my hiking companions—grew tired, it occurred to me that we might not get to the mouth of the canyon before dark. At about 5:00 p.m., we reached an impasse along the creek-side route through which we had been bushwhacking. The creek tumbled over a ten-foot drop we could not negotiate. And there, at the bottom of the canyon, we had no cell-phone reception.

In a last attempt to find a pathway out of the canyon, we decided to climb the steep northern wall where, if we failed to find a way out, at least we could get a signal to call for help. Once it was clear that we could not hike out before dark, we dialed 911.

Davis County Search and Rescue initially tried to reach us with ATVs, but we were too far up the canyon. Because I started cramping as the temperature cooled in the gathering dusk, we were unable to hike to where the vehicles could climb.

Faced with that dilemma, the rescuers sent for a helicopter just before dark. Amazingly, the pilot set one of the landing struts of his craft on a flat-topped rock the size of a living room chair about fifty yards from where I stood. He managed to hold the helicopter steady while his assistant jumped to the ground, found me, and assisted me back to the flat-topped rock.

My spasming legs were close to useless, so I leaned heavily on the rescuer as I half walked and was half hauled to the waiting, roaring helicopter. Between the crew and Hillary, I was pushed and pulled into the helicopter, which then flew to a meetinghouse owned by The Church of Jesus Christ of Latter-day Saints in Bountiful. In the parking lot, I received medical attention in an ambulance. After being warmed and receiving IV-fluid resuscitation, I was judged well enough to be released to go home.

Before leaving for home, I asked my attendants how much the rescue services would cost and whether I could be billed for them. The reply startled me. There would be no bill. Davis County Search and Rescue never charged for the assistance it rendered—even in a case like mine where my mistakes had caused the problem. Their policy was simple: they did not want people in difficulty to be so concerned about the cost that they failed to call for help.

Because of that experience, City Creek Canyon has come to symbolize one aspect of health-system reform for me. When we as a society decide to tax ourselves to pay for health care (or helicopter rescue), we are merely doing what makes sense. People are not isolated. We depend on each other, help each other, and induce our government to organize and fund services for all. Life, liberty, and the pursuit of happiness (including a late-spring hike in City Creek Canyon), the quintessential American values, all require that we be in good health—and are educated, have paved roads, are protected by police and fire services, and are defended by the military, among other things.

Our taxes have funded gigantic improvements in the care of the sick and injured during the past century. We build hospitals, organize emergency services, train doctors and nurses, and design treatments and vaccines with public funds. After taxing ourselves more heavily for health care than any other citizenry in the world, it is absurd that, unlike my experience with Davis County Search and Rescue, millions of Americans cannot pursue life, liberty, and happiness because they cannot afford necessary illness and injury care.

The most common cause of personal bankruptcy in the United States is debt related to illness or injury care. And most of those bankrupted by healthcare costs had health insurance at the time they suffered expensive illness or injury. The business model of American-style health financing is all about optimal profit, making health insurance useless either as a guarantor of financial security or payer and organizer for needed health care.

Despite its uselessness, however, health insurance—whether a benefit of employment or an offering of the Affordable Care Act —is itself subsidized by the taxes and tax policies of the United States government. Paradoxically, the leaders of American health insurance both lobby for increasing taxation for revenues to support public healthcare financing and argue that publicly financed health care is "socialism" and should therefore be opposed. It is well past time for all of us to stop listening to the self-serving rhetoric of the health-insurance profiteers.

Each time I'm in City Creek Canyon, and I run there several times each week, I remember the helicopter crew dispatched at public expense to rescue me from a threatening situation. And each time, I am reminded that we Americans need to shed our fear of "socialized" medicine and recognize public funding of health care for what it is: a gift we can give ourselves. So, let's reserve that gift—public revenues for the direct funding of necessary healthcare services—for the people of the United States of America themselves and stop allowing those funds to pass through for-profit insurance corporations that provide us with neither financial security nor high-quality, efficiently financed health care. A regionally cooperative healthcare system with unified public financing is the best way to accomplish that goal.

And let's take a hard look at the dollars involved. The cost of care in other first-world countries is *nothing* like that of the United States, where prices are outrageous. In the United States, health goods and services are commonly ten times higher (or more!) than elsewhere in the developed world.

Why?

Simple: in the United States, we pretend that market forces are effective in distributing medicine and surgery. We Americans seem to share the common belief that market forces will somehow magically bring rising healthcare costs under control. That has never been true, and it still isn't. Economist and mathematician Kenneth Arrow won a Nobel Prize in economics sixty years ago for describing how market forces fail to function in healthcare delivery. But Americans, unlike the citizens of every other first-world country, continue to stubbornly try to fit the square peg of market competition into the round hole of health care.

The prerequisites for optimal competitive market function have been known since 1776, when Adam Smith published *The Wealth of Nations*. Buyers must be able to know for themselves all about the products and services for which they "shop"; sellers must have no other interest than in making the best deal possible for themselves; transactions in the market must not have meaning or implications for anyone other than the buyer and the seller;

and there must be an inverse relationship between price and demand.

None of these prerequisites are true of healthcare delivery in the United States. Look at how Adam Smith's prerequisites stack up in today's American healthcare system:

- First, buyers can't shop because they are patients, not consumers; they are sick, sometimes incapacitated. They don't know what they need or how to recognize good quality in health care.
- Second, sellers of health care, like doctors and nurses, are under an ethical obligation to place their patients' needs before their own interests.
- Third, every healthcare transaction has implications for everyone else in the community, whether treating a case of infectious tuberculosis or making sure that trauma-care providers are constantly able to "practice" their craft.
- Finally, demand for healthcare goods and services is *not* determined by price. It's determined by epidemiology and the frequency of disease and injury. No one ever buys an appendectomy because it is on sale.

Americans have an important decision to make. Do we want to continue with business as usual, making the insurance companies and other medical corporations (aka the medical-industrial complex) richer by the day at the expense of patients who often cannot afford the care they need? Or do we want to prioritize patients over profits?

It's a very simple decision, really. And the wellness of all depends on how we answer.

2

AVARICE VERSUS ALTRUISM

E ven the wealthiest American would be financially unable to maintain today's highly intense services at the ready should they find themselves in need of urgent care like I did near City Creek Canyon. For example, there are only seventy-seven accredited burn-care centers in the United States verified by the American Burn Association. Salt Lake City is home to one of these centers, which is located at the University of Utah Medical Center. It is one of the few burn-care centers in the entire Intermountain region, which includes large parts of Idaho, Montana, Wyoming, Colorado, Arizona, Nevada, and all of Utah. Tourists who accidentally fall in and are scalded by the thermal features at Yellowstone National Park often end up in the burn unit at the University of Utah Medical Center, no matter where in the world they actually live.

Burn care is extraordinarily expensive. The average survivor of a major burn injury spends two weeks in the ICU and almost four weeks in the hospital, usually with months of therapy thereafter. The total average cost for a major burn injury is around $200,000. As hefty as that amount is, it is possible that the hospitals that host burn centers end up losing money on that specific enterprise. Salaries, supplies, training, and the costs of maintaining everything at the ready for the moment of a burn injury are enormous. Billionaire fortunes are not enough to maintain the expense of that readiness, in part because billionaires have the means to travel all over the country and would therefore need to assure the availability of burn care (and other emergency services) throughout the nation. It takes all of us together to pay for the care we might need in the eventuality of significant injury or illness.

There is a corollary to this City Creek Canyon metaphor for health-system reform. The canyon serves up another touchpoint in my personal history that has become part of the origins of my opinions about how to reform American health care. When Brigham Young first led a group of Latter-day Saint pioneers into the Salt Lake Valley, City Creek emerged from its canyon and traversed the northern portion of the valley in a westerly direction until merging with the Jordan River before eventually emptying into the Great Salt Lake. Brigham established his household on the banks of the creek and diverted water from it for his family garden.

Long before I first lived in Salt Lake City, however, the creek bed outside the canyon on the valley floor had disappeared under urban construction and the flow of water was directed into underground conduits. By the early 1980s, when I initially lived in the area, Salt Lake Valley residents had all but forgotten that the perennial flow of water from City Creek Canyon had been buried. So it was a puzzle to me one Sunday morning in late May 1983 when I drove up Second Avenue heading east from the intersection of State Street and North Temple in downtown Salt Lake City and encountered a small but growing stream of water flowing from City Creek Canyon toward the city center.

That Sunday morning, I was en route to the Salt Lake Veterans Administration Medical Center, where I was serving the final month of my internship in family practice. By the time I finished my rounds a couple of hours later, the small but growing stream of water I had observed that morning had become a flood that completely blocked traffic on the west end of the Avenues.

This flood occurred because the underground conduit into which City Creek usually flowed became clogged with mud, rocks, and debris, causing the creek to jump its banks. Flow in the creek on that day in 1983 was three and a half times the flood stage and twice as high as the previous, 1921 record for spring runoff. The unusually high water flow in 1983 was due to a winter snowpack 50 percent higher than normal, and cool temperatures into late May had prevented any earlier melt. The resulting massive rapid snowmelt inundated City Creek Canyon and resulted in a four-foot flow of water onto State Street for two weeks.

Buildings along State Street were saved from catastrophe by six thousand volunteers who filled and placed one million sandbags during fifty-thousand-person days of effort. The business owners in Salt Lake City with some of the priciest business locations in Utah were saved from devastation by the unpaid efforts of average Utahns who came to help because they were needed, never expecting any compensation. Altruism is a powerful but often under-recognized economic force. Human beings are not best served by unfettered self-interest. Altruism is the highest expression of human character and best fosters creativity and caring. Altruism is how we maintain our societal structure and cohesion.

U.S. citizens are currently laboring under the illusion that only the for-profit motive can sustain the growth of anything of value in medical care. As an example, while serving as the Nevada state health officer in 1989, I remember listening to a physician/business leader touting the importance of the for-profit business model in the delivery of health care. He was the CEO of the largest HMO in the Silver State during my tenure as the public-health leader in the late 1980s, and he was fond of saying that nonprofit healthcare institutions were not accountable to anyone because they had no stockholders and were therefore not functioning optimally. Of course, he failed to mention that as the CEO of a for-profit HMO, his accountability to the owners of that enterprise was simply to make as much money as possible for them. In contrast, he had no fiduciary duty to the members or patients of the HMO to provide the best healthcare services with the best possible efficiency. As one of the principal regulators of that HMO, I can attest that it often failed its members in health-care quality and efficiency, even though it was very profitable. On one occasion, that HMO failed to arrange for the care of newborns in a hospital in Carson City, Nevada. On another, the members or patients who had paid the premiums for health coverage from that HMO were denied ENT or orthopedic specialty services. But the lack of care for patients was of no consequence to an HMO CEO seeking to pad the quarterly bottom line for his investors.

Americans have the most profitable healthcare system in the world, yet American patients are least likely in the first world to benefit from proven mortality-reducing medical interventions. For example, in the United States, insulin therapy on average now costs up to $400 per month, which is five to nine times more expensive than elsewhere in the developed world. High prices for insulin and other pharmaceuticals in this country are common because the for-profit pharmaceutical industry in the United States has as its principal objective the maximum enrichment of its stockholders, not the care of patients needing medication. Diabetic patients may suffer life-threatening illness if unable to afford insulin, but the officers of a for-profit pharmaceutical firm have no fiduciary duty to care about whether diabetic patients live or die.

Many apologists for the for-profit motive in health care argue that pharmaceutical firms are merely charging what the "market" will bear. I believe what they mean by this is that under normal circumstances, prices in a market economy are regulated by demand. In a functioning market, if a seller prices goods and services too high, demand falls and prices are driven down. As prices subsequently fall, demand increases. This central tenet of market theory maintains that demand is inversely proportional to price.

That's total nonsense when it comes to insulin, which sells at a remarkably high price in the United States. Insulin is not a product that is in demand because of its price. The vast majority of Americans, those who do not have diabetes and therefore do not need insulin, would not acquire insulin even if it were given away without charge. No price is low enough to drive demand for insulin if you are not diabetic.

Conversely, if you *do* have insulin-dependent diabetes and your life depends on purchasing it, no price is too high to dissuade you from trying to buy it. Demand for insulin is not driven by its price. Demand for insulin is driven by how often the disease process of diabetes takes hold in people's lives; with increasing numbers of people with diabetes will come increasing demand for insulin. Market economics has nothing to do with it.

In order to hide their true motive, apologists for the for-profit motive in health care pretend that market economics apply to healthcare delivery. That motive is to harvest windfall profits from the sick, injured, and dying patients of the United States— and to fleece the healthy as often as possible through the payment of premiums while receiving, in turn, as little promise for care as the health-insurance company can get away with.

The current high cost of insulin in the United States is an historical irony. It has been a century since insulin was first purified enough to use in the care of diabetes mellitus. Working in a lab at the University of Toronto, Frederick Banting and Charles Best first published the results of their research isolating insulin from the pancreas of dogs and then using it to successfully reduce the blood sugar of diabetic dogs in November 1921. With the help of others, they purified bovine insulin and began treating human diabetics in 1922.

The collaborators decided to transfer the patent rights for their insulin purification process to the University of Toronto so that no third party could secure a profitable monopoly and they could guarantee quality control in the use of the patent. Banting, Best, and their colleagues sold their valuable, lifesaving technology to their host institution for a dollar, which they considered the ethically correct step to take. They intended that no diabetic patient should be priced out of access to insulin.

As recent American experience proves, Banting and Best were right to be worried about avarice interrupting diabetic patient care. And their original intention—that no diabetic patient be priced out of access to insulin—eventually went unrealized as insulin, now part of a competitive pharmaceutical industry, skyrocketed in price.

Let's take a hard look at what has happened to the price of insulin. U.S. Senator Ron Wyden of Oregon said of the pharmaceutical industry as a whole, "The pharmaceutical pricing system is just rigged, and it's rigged so patients pay more each year. Competition does not drive prices down."[1]

That's especially true for insulin, said Wyden, who co-led a two-year bipartisan investigation into insulin prices. The committee examined internal documents from the three largest insulin manufacturers—Eli Lilly, Sanofi, and Novo Nordisk—as well as from the three largest pharmacy benefit managers (PBMs), the middleman companies who negotiate contracts with the drug companies.

"What our investigation found is that the [PBMs] actually have a financial incentive to keep prices high," reported Wyden. The investigation also concluded that drug companies "aggressively" raised the list prices—the amount manufacturers set for their products—even in the absence of "significant advances in the efficacy of the drugs."[2]

The result is that patients pay substantially more each year for insulin. And the fallout? According to the American Diabetes Association, an estimated 650,000 insulin-dependent diabetics in this country are rationing insulin—a drug they need to survive—because of cost.

In the case of diabetes, that's a life-or-death dilemma. When a young, divorced mother was recently unable to afford insulin on her salary and did not have access to health insurance because of her part-time status, she had to stop using it. Her death—and the deaths of many in similar situations—is a stark condemnation of how greed has overcome the important charge of protecting patient health. And she wasn't the only one forced by circumstances to stop taking essential medication: upon her death, her young son was returned to his abusive father, a situation that had caused the divorce to begin with.

More importantly, Banting and Best illustrate the power of altruism as a motive for creativity and care in medicine. The for-profit, self-serving motive fails in comparison to altruism in attracting optimal efforts to improve care by the best and brightest minds. When used nearly exclusively as the model for healthcare delivery, as is currently the case in the United States, the for-profit motive also skews the actions of individuals and organizations away from what patients truly need.

Perhaps the greatest pharmaceutical innovation needed today is new kinds of antibiotics. Without new antibiotics, organisms that are resistant to treatment—such as methicillin-resistant *Staphylococcus aureus* (MRSA), penicillin-resistant *Enterococcus*, and multidrug-resistant *Mycobacterium tuberculosis* (MDR-TB)—will increasingly threaten the lives of patients worldwide.

One woman in her early sixties became infected with *Enterococcus* through a small sore located in an area that completely escaped her attention. Though she felt fine when she awakened in the morning, by early evening, her worried family members had taken her to the emergency room, where she was found to be incoherent with a fever of almost 110 degrees. The infection had become systemic, overwhelming her body's ability to fight it off.

She was admitted to the intensive care unit with a less-than-optimistic prognosis: the *Enterococcus* was resistant to the antibiotics in the hospital's arsenal, and doctors were uncertain whether they could save her. Over the next two weeks, a team of infectious-disease specialists and other physicians worked tirelessly, trying various combinations of medications and procedures to combat the woman's sepsis. After more than three weeks in the hospital—a period during which two other patients in the ICU died from antibiotic-resistant sepsis—she was able to go home with a PICC line (a long, flexible tube inserted into a vein through which medications are given) and continued on antibiotics for seven weeks. She was unable to return to her regular activities for almost three months due to the lingering ravages of her infection.

The devastation of antibiotic-resistant infection affects people of all ages and from all walks of life. A man in his thirties lost his leg to a resistant strain of *Staphylococcus* after almost a month in the hospital. Another in his fifties developed MRSA and progressed from being totally healthy to dying in a hospital only five days later from the infection doctors were unable to treat with their arsenal of existing antibiotics.

These are only a few examples of what has become all too common. Each year in the United States, 2.8 million patients get an antibiotic-resistant infection, and more than 35,000 of them die. Yet it has only been within the last year that a consortium of private organizations catalyzed by public funds announced a concerted effort to bring new antibiotics to patients within the coming decade.

When I am in City Creek Canyon today, I think of helicopters and floods, and I remember that what is needed in American health care is a renewal of our national commitment to give ourselves the gift of health care so that each American can be optimally healthy and best able to pursue life, liberty, and happiness. In order to sustainably give that gift to ourselves, Americans need to eschew the for-profit model in medicine, particularly the business model of American health insurers. And we need to stop allowing the health insurers and others who are profiting at the expense of the sick and injured to label the public funding of health care as "socialized medicine."

The pejorative use of the term *socialism* is intended to obscure the true nature of how health care is already funded and how it would be best and most efficiently managed for American patients, as discussed in chapter 1. We tax ourselves to build American infrastructure because that's what is sensible and practical in supporting the life, liberty, and pursuit of happiness for all Americans. I have never heard our interstate highways called the "socialized streets of America."

You probably think it's counterintuitive for me to write from the point of view of a conservative while espousing government-funded, nonprofit health-system reform. I do so because it is my contention that state-based health-system reform featuring regionally cooperative private-sector care delivery with unified public financing is the only viable conservative approach to improving American health-system function.

Health care is often presented as a very partisan issue. Americans have become accustomed to hearing the Republican Party oppose anything other than private, for-profit, market-based healthcare delivery. But even though that party supposedly espouses conservative values, that's *not* a conservative health policy because it is federally based, extremely expensive and therefore fiscally irresponsible, and careless toward human life and health while careful to cater to the requirements of special interests. And Republicans aren't the only ones who support this health policy. The Democratic Party also supports a "market-based" health policy and is therefore equally to blame for the corporate rip-off that so characterizes the American medical-industrial complex. In other words, the two sides are actually closely aligned in making sure that the *money* is what's important —not the health and welfare of the people.

Both parties share the responsibility—and the blame. The Affordable Care Act (also known as Obamacare) is a case in point. It seems many Americans see Obamacare as a responsible, altruistic, generous system. In reality, though, it's meant to line insurers' pockets. Unlike the purpose of Congressional action outlined in the U.S. Constitution, to promote the general welfare, this Democrat-passed health statute enriched corporate America at the expense of Americans most in need. As an example of the enormous revenues realized through Obamacare, consider the profitability of just one major health insurer. When Mr. Biden was sworn in as vice president in 2009, a share of United Health stock cost $21.55. Twelve years later, the day he was sworn in as president of the United States, that same share was worth $350.84—a *sixteenfold increase in value*.

Coming in second as a federally legislated source of corporate health profiteering is the Republican-passed Part D of Medicare, which uses taxpayer money to purchase pharmaceuticals for senior citizens. In the course of making these purchases, Medicare Part D, as explicitly written and implemented by the Republicans, forbids the federal government from negotiating with the pharmaceutical industry for best prices. *How on earth did this happen?* Patients are left in the dust when it comes to getting their medications for a better price. This policy has directly led to the abuses of the faux market for pharmaceuticals, as illustrated by the price of insulin.

The Affordable Care Act and Medicare Part D are egregious examples of federal legislation catering to corporate profiteers and failing to provide a commensurate increase in value for the American patient. Patients in the United States receive mediocre care (the poorest quality in the developed world) that is inefficiently financed (overhead in the United States wastes $500 billion a year), all at a ridiculously high price because inefficient, poor-quality care costs more. The only real objective of business as usual in American health care is to make as much profit as possible.

And this is important to understand: the problem doesn't rest with just one party. With *both* parties competing to consent to the profiteering interests of the medical-industrial complex, neither the principles of the progressive movement within the Democratic Party nor the traditional tried-and-true Republican principles of conservatism are reflected in how the United States currently does business when it comes to health care. It's not a contest between parties; it's the politicians versus the people.

There is only one accurate description of a healthcare system that profits excessively by harming patients—*avaricious*. Avarice is not a conservative value. Protecting the interests of greedy business enterprises should not be the object of conservative politicians. On this point, I agree with Adam Smith, the conservative's iconic original market theorist, who authored *The Wealth of Nations* in 1776. In *The Theory of Moral Sentiments*, Smith said:

> "The great source of both the misery and disorders of human life, seems to arise from over-rating the difference between one permanent situation and another. Avarice over-rates the difference between poverty and riches: ambition, that between a private and a public station: vain-glory, that between obscurity and extensive reputation. The person under the influence of any of those extravagant passions, is not only miserable in his actual situation, but is often disposed to disturb the peace of society, in order to arrive at that which he so foolishly admires. The slightest observation, however, might satisfy him, that, in all the ordinary situations of human life, a well-disposed mind may be equally calm, equally cheerful, and equally contented.

Some of those situations may, no doubt, deserve to be preferred to others: but none of them can deserve to be pursued with that passionate ardor which drives us to violate the rules either of prudence or of justice; or to corrupt the future tranquility of our minds, either by shame from the remembrance of our own folly, or by remorse from the horror of our own injustice."

Both political parties have been disturbing the peace of American society for much of the past three decades. But Republicans have been most especially responsible for the violation of the rules of prudence and justice, resulting in the corruption of tranquility during the years of the Trump administration. With the emergence of the progressive wing of the Democratic party, there is now a challenge from the left taking on the avaricious corporation-entrenched Democratic politics of the past three decades. However, frankly, there has not been strong conservatism in American politics for some time, at least as that term was understood by Abraham Lincoln, who asked, "What is conservatism? Is it not the adherence to the old and tried against the new and untried?" Note that Mr. Lincoln would not have included allegiance to party within his definition of "adherence to the old and tried," since he left his original political party, the Whig Party, to join a brand-new political organization, which became the Grand Old Party (the GOP, or Republican).

Ultimately, original conservatism was focused on the welfare of all people, recognizing that some needed more help than others, but everyone was a contributor to the success of the American experiment. Patriotism was not allegiance to party or politician but a genuine interest in policy and action that addressed any problems facing the country.

The leaders of conservatism found strength and wisdom in the Bible as an original source of truth but allowed each citizen the right to believe whatever best suited the individual without allowing religious tenets to control the policy of the government. On the other hand, the rule of law was an absolute; no exceptions were allowed, not even for the denizen of the White House. As the United States grew into its destined size and economic power, conservative American leaders recognized the absolute necessity of an international role for their country in the pursuit of world peace and prosperity. That is the original conservatism that surrounded me and informed my understanding as a young child during the Eisenhower administration.

3

STATE-BASED HEALTH REFORM: WHAT CONSERVATIVES BELIEVE

I was born in Tucson, Arizona, during Eisenhower's first term. By the time his second term ended, I was old enough to notice and be interested in the televised Kennedy/Nixon debates. I remember my early childhood as a time of relative peace and prosperity devoid of political rancor. Kennedy's ascension to the presidency, while not embraced enthusiastically by most of the adults I knew, was nonetheless no cause for alarm, even though he won by the narrowest of margins (which Richard Nixon did not challenge, saying later that people needed to know who their president would be). Differences of opinion were never characterized as cataclysmic harbingers of national doom. No one believed that an electoral loss would lead to the imminent demise of the American way of life.

The dominant political force during my childhood and adolescence in suburban Phoenix was Barry Goldwater's conservatism. In general, Goldwater embraced the principles of original conservatism propagated by Lincoln, Grant, Roosevelt, and Eisenhower. Like them, Goldwater believed what Theodore Roosevelt had so aptly stated, "This country will not be a permanently good place for any of us to live in unless we make it a reasonably good place for all of us to live in."[1]

Goldwater was at the forefront of desegregation efforts in Arizona at his business, in schools, in the military, and in civic affairs. When elected to the United States Senate, he desegregated its lunchroom, insisting that his African American assistant be served there like anyone else who worked in the Congressional offices. He agonized over his vote against the Civil Rights Act of 1964 but felt justified in that vote because the act, he believed, centralized too much power in the hands of the federal government and therefore pitted two of his founding principles against each other—racial equality and the Tenth Amendment. Later in life, he admitted that his vote against the Civil Rights Act of 1964 was his preeminent regret. He was a lifelong member of the NAACP (the National Association for the Advancement of Colored People).

Barry Goldwater considered himself a friend of President Kennedy, and as he plotted his political course in the early 1960s, he thought he might garner the Republican presidential nomination in 1964 and then travel the country with Kennedy, debating the issues. But with the assassination of Kennedy came the presidency of Lyndon Johnson, precluding the opportunity for a gentle campaign contest between two friends. It was simply inconceivable to Goldwater that anyone would gin up political support by asserting that an opponent's victory would be the end of the country—but President Johnson did exactly that to Goldwater in 1964.

Barry Goldwater was an original American conservative, perhaps one of only three in the post-Cold War Era (I include later Republican presidential nominees John McCain and Mitt Romney in this group). Goldwater was fully on board with his Republican predecessors in his faith in the individual citizen. He said:

"We Americans understand freedom; we have earned it, we have lived for it, and we have died for it. This nation and its people are freedom's models in a searching world. We can be freedom's missionaries in a doubting world. The genius of the American system is that through freedom we have created extraordinary results from plain old ordinary people."[2]

He also acknowledged the importance of biblical values as underpinnings in American society, stating:

"Conservatism, we are told, is out-of-date. This charge is preposterous, and we ought to boldly say so. The laws of God, and of nature, have no dateline. . . . These principles are derived from the nature of man, and from the truths that God has revealed about His creation. . . . To suggest that the Conservative philosophy is out of date is akin to saying that the Golden Rule, or the Ten Commandments or Aristotle's Politics are out of date."[3]

Goldwater, however, did not accept that the tenets of religious denominations should come to dominate political discourse or dictate the policies of government. He said, "I am a conservative Republican, but I believe in democracy and the separation of church and state. The conservative movement is founded on the simple tenet that people have the right to live life as they please as long as they don't hurt anyone else in the process."[4]

He further stated, "The great decisions of government cannot be dictated by the concerns of religious factions. . . . We have succeeded for 205 years in keeping the affairs of state separate from the uncompromising idealism of religious groups and we mustn't stop now. To retreat from that separation would violate the principles of conservatism and the values upon which the framers built this democratic republic."[5]

He was emphatic when it came to the effects of religious zeal on the political process:

> "I can say with conviction that the religious issues of these groups have little or nothing to do with conservative or liberal politics. The uncompromising position of these groups is a divisive element that could tear apart the very spirit of our representative system, if they gain sufficient strength. As it is, they are diverting us away from the vital issues that our Government needs to address. Far too much of the time of members of Congress and officials in the Executive Branch is used up dealing with special-interest groups on issues like abortion, school busing, ERA, prayer in the schools and pornography. While these are important moral issues, they are secondary right now to our national security and economic survival."[6]

Goldwater was a pro-choice conservative, a position he believed to be inherently logical and integrated. About the treatment of our gay fellow citizens, he simply said, "You don't need to be straight to fight and die for your country. You just need to shoot straight."[7]

Goldwater joined Teddy Roosevelt in the modern conservative interest in conservation, saying, "While I am a great believer in the free enterprise system and all that it entails, I am an even stronger believer in the right of our people to live in a clean and pollution-free environment."[8]

But for Goldwater, the policy arena deserving the best efforts of original conservatives in the post-Cold War Era was the growth of the federal government and its increasing reach into the lives of individual Americans. In essence, the debate was about the meaning of the American Constitution, of which Goldwater maintained, "The constitution is an instrument, above all, for limiting the functions of government."[9]

Barry Goldwater held that conservatism would end if it failed to find and articulate a line of demarcation that limited the reach of the federal government. I believe he was correct about that. Original American conservatism no longer exists as a viable force in American politics precisely because members of today's Republican party are not consistent about limiting what the federal government should do or how each branch of the federal government should interact.

"We the People of the United States," reads the Preamble to the Constitution, "in Order to form a more perfect Union, establish Justice, insure domestic Tranquility, provide for the common defence, promote the general Welfare, and secure the Blessings of Liberty to ourselves and our Posterity, do ordain and establish this Constitution for the United States of America." American government has a role to play in organizing unity, justice, peace, security, welfare, and freedom. These are, therefore, conservative, constitutional values. But exactly how American government should go about playing this role—specifically what level of American government should assume responsibility for these various essential functions—is the subject of the articles of and amendments to the Constitution.

Goldwater articulated that the rule of law in the United States limited the functions of the federal government and protected the role of state government when concerned with issues of promoting the general welfare, such as dealing with unemployment, the care of the sick and injured, and other human-services issues. Today's so-called conservatives have abandoned the debates about how and through what level of government the general welfare should be promoted. Busied as they are with the uncompromising "idealism" of religious groups and with the special interests that feed on the nation in times of peace and conspire against it in times of adversity, today's Republicans feign conservatism and have ceased to be interested in the old-and-tried values of original American conservatism. And so, in

Barry Goldwater's words, "Conservatism is through."[10] It has ceased to exist as a force for good in American governance.

The best demonstration of the demise of conservatism in America is the mangled mess Congress has made of health policy. Republicans and Democrats, as already noted, are both to blame for the pitiful state of American health care, which is characterized by massive cost caused by poor quality and inefficiency. Members of both parties sanctimoniously scream at each other about absurdities such as "death panels" (supposed committees of doctors or bureaucrats who decide which patients get treatment and which are left to die), "socialism," "access," and "coverage." In the meantime, both parties espouse the world's highest healthcare taxes to enrich corporations at the expense of the sick and dying. Members of Congress from both parties pass federal budgets and bills, while administrations from both parties issue executive orders and regulations that federalize health policy without ever considering the primacy of the Tenth Amendment.

Eisenhower rightly warned that the military-industrial complex would threaten our liberties and democracy—but today, the *medical*-industrial complex is robbing us of both our current health and our nation's future economic vitality. We are rightly warned that money power in the country will endeavor to prolong its reign by working upon the prejudices of the people until all wealth is aggregated in a few hands, which will lead to the destruction of our American way of governance. What an apt description of business as usual in American healthcare delivery.

Teddy Roosevelt warned a century ago about business interests corrupting politics:

> "Our government, National and State, must be freed from the sinister influence or control of special interests. Exactly as the special interests of cotton and slavery threatened our political integrity before the Civil War, so now the great special business

interests too often control and corrupt the men and methods of government for their own profit. We must drive the special interests out of politics."[11]

The absence of original conservatism in the current body politic of the United States has ripened the corruption of our healthcare system. Without anyone articulating the original conservative values in today's health-policy debates, there has been no countervailing force applied against the avarice of corporate interests.

What was true of politics in the Gilded Age just prior to Theodore Roosevelt's presidency is again true today. "The old parties are husks," he said, "with no real soul within either, divided on artificial lines, boss-ridden and privilege-controlled, each a jumble of incongruous elements, and neither daring to speak out wisely and fearlessly on what should be said on the vital issues of the day."[12]

I believe the GOP lost its soul to powerful corporate interests, most especially the medical-industrial complex. The pretense that market forces will solve all health-system troubles is the hollow core of Republican domestic policy. Year after year, Republicans have voted to heavily tax Americans for health care. Today's total annual funding for health care is over $4 trillion; this includes funding for Medicare, Medicaid, CHIP, Obamacare supplements, military and civil-service health benefits, tax credits for employer health benefits, plus an acronym soup of other state and federal health programs. Americans are the most taxed citizenry in the world when it comes to health care, yet the middle class and those even less well-off can't afford to care for their families when sick or injured. Financing health care is a challenge even for the upper middle class.

President Biden's election is, in my opinion, the symbolic end of the soul of his party because it kills any pretense that the Democratic Party is anything other than a slave to corporate interests, especially the medical-industrial complex. The rising reaction, weak as it is, from the progressive wing of the Democratic Party against the corporation-oriented Biden administration illustrates this point.

Health-system reform is the sentinel domestic issue of our time. Massive governmental spending on health care threatens the fiscal solvency of our nation, our state governments, and our families. The opportunity cost of that massive spending has eroded public education and our national infrastructure. Poor-quality health care threatens our lives, and the preference for sales over care enslaves millions more to medications, addictions, unnecessary surgeries, and other interventions. Poor patient safety practices in American hospitals lead to the premature deaths of hundreds of thousands of people. We are served poorly by a healthcare system that gets clinically proven care done correctly only about half the time.

Obamacare, which Biden famously and vulgarly called "a big deal," makes all that is bad about American health care worse because it, too, worships the false idol of marketized medicine. Obamacare is the culmination of the transformation of the Democratic Party from an institution that historically tried to find a way to care for all Americans to its modern-day status as a political party that cares most for corporations. Democrats, like Republicans, have for decades voted to satisfy any demand from the medical-industrial complex at the expense of American families and patients. This seems to be an obvious violation of what historically mattered to Democrats, though I admittedly view it from outside their party. Franklin D. Roosevelt and Harry Truman both proposed universal health care, and Lyndon B. Johnson led the nation to Medicare and Medicaid. Jimmy Carter, the legitimate current spokesman for the soul of the Democratic Party, has said that better, simpler, and therefore cheaper care with regionally cooperative private-sector healthcare delivery and unified, public financing is (or should be) the future of American health policy. Why hasn't President Biden listened to Mr. Carter?

Progressivism, invented by Teddy Roosevelt, is no longer a Republican concept, and healthcare progress no longer exists in the soul of the Democratic Party. Mr. Biden is taking the Democratic Party further down the corporate rathole and thereby losing the support of millions of progressive party members. These two soulless political parties force American voters to witness recurrent pointless rounds of partisan bickering about Obamacare instead of engaging in real discussion about the facts of American health care gone awry.

For example, Medicaid expansion under the so-called Affordable Care Act has been implemented in thirty-seven states; most of the gains in "coverage" under Obamacare have come through this expansion. Proponents of Medicaid expansion argue that all people deserve care when sick or injured and that Medicaid can finance that care for people whose incomes are too low to afford care on their own. Opponents of Medicaid expansion, obviously including the majority of "red state" legislatures and governors, argue that Medicaid costs are rising faster than GDP growth, an unsustainable trend both for state and federal governments.

Both sides are partly right. People of all economic strata are healthier if they are blessed with some means of financing needed health care, but healthcare costs are exploding in the United States, and it is irresponsible to ignore that reality. Thus, we have a perpetual, unresolvable, partisan divide about health-system reform, specifically the variation of reform known as Obamacare.

Both sides are ignoring the overwhelming evidence about what is wrong with their own point of view. Proponents of Obamacare are ignoring the fact that Obamacare has failed as a coverage initiative, leaving tens of millions of Americans without healthcare financing even before tens of millions more lost job-related health benefits during the COVID-19 pandemic. It is manifestly unfair to tax a populace for the healthcare costs of those too poor to pay taxes while the middle-class taxpayers are at substantial risk of insolvency if they encounter a significant illness or injury. And the American taxpayer was already paying the highest tax burden for health care *before* the Affordable Care Act was passed. "Coverage" expansion is not the health-system reform needed.

Beyond failing as a coverage initiative, Obamacare fails at both protecting patients and being affordable despite its title. Some 250,000 deaths occur in the United States each year due to preventable injury of hospitalized patients, a shocking statistic to which Obamacare has no answer. No patients are protected by Obamacare, nor is it affordable, either for families or the government. And, as mentioned earlier, recent data documented that two-thirds of families in the United States are driven to bankruptcy by illness and injury costs—even though most of these families had health insurance. Employment-based health benefits no longer provide financial security for Americans who face significant illness or injury.

The opponents of Obamacare are wrong to assume that market-oriented strategies will correct what's wrong with American healthcare delivery. For instance, the implementation of health savings accounts and high-deductible health plans has hollowed out health benefits, leading to financial disaster for American patients. And market-oriented strategies don't deal with quality-of-care issues, such as patient injury.

It's time for us to stop bickering about Obamacare. These pointless arguments don't address the real issue: cost. Americans outspend the citizens of every other developed nation in health care by a wide margin. American health care costs too much because of quality waste and inefficiency. Poor-quality care, including poor patient safety practices, amounts to $700 billion per year in quality waste. Dependence on the private, for-profit health insurance business model, with its incredibly high overheads, leads to an additional $500 billion per year in inefficiency waste.

Health-system reform featuring better, simpler care through regionally cooperative private-sector healthcare delivery and unified public financing, studied dozens of times in recent years, offers the cost savings needed for sustainable reform. It's time to stop debating Obamacare, take a cue from Barry Goldwater, and start talking about how to make it possible for one or more states to implement better private-sector care with simpler public-sector health financing. While running as a first-time candidate for the United States Senate in 2010, Senator Mike Lee (R-UT) stated that he would support federal legislation to allow state-based better and simpler health-system reform. We voters should be calling on Senator Lee, who, characteristically, hasn't lifted a finger to solve his constituents' healthcare problems, and all his Senate colleagues to make good on that campaign promise, because I am tired of the nonsense that passes for political discourse in this country.

For example, the candidates for the U.S. House of Representatives from Utah's 4th Congressional District in 2018 met for a "debate." During one excruciating segment, both these esteemed persons, each holding an important office at the time, repeatedly took swipes at one another over the federal deficit without ever mentioning the most important cause of federal debt—healthcare spending. (Federal revenues are projected to keep up with future federal outlays for all categories of spending with the exception of our massive healthcare programs, including Medicare, Medicaid, CHIP, and others.)

Not long after exchanging meaningless sentiments about federal debt, the two candidates were actually asked about health care. Again, they failed to address the real issues, choosing instead to snipe endlessly at each other over whether Obamacare should be salvaged or repealed. These two candidates either didn't know or didn't care about the basic facts concerning our nation's single most important domestic issue: our massively wasteful, generally dysfunctional healthcare system. Wouldn't it be refreshing if the electorate could actually hear candidates articulating the real issues and proposing real solutions?

But this is our own fault. We, the voters of America, who repeatedly opine that we dislike Congress nonetheless put up with campaign drivel and generally reelect our own member of Congress. Let's change this. We deserve better. If you care about health-system reform, make a judgment about the candidates running for Congress in your district; determine who will best serve American patients without regard to the political party they represent. Voters concerned about health-system reform should begin each election cycle with a bias against incumbents since those incumbents have manifestly already failed to change business as usual in our healthcare system.

I challenge every American voter to reach out to the candidates for Congress during the coming election cycle and tell them what you want them to do about health-system reform. For those of you puzzled about what you should demand from Congress, here are some facts and ideas:

- Americans pay the world's highest taxes for health care. Two-thirds of our nation's more than $4 trillion annual health spending comes from the taxpayer. Every other first-world nation spends far less and has better health outcomes. The American healthcare system, compared to those of other first-world nations, wastes $1 trillion per year in healthcare spending because of poor-quality care and inefficiency.
- "Coverage" programs like Obamacare are not health-system reform. No one needs health insurance, which is the world's most useless, wasteful, expensive health-financing scheme.

- What every American needs is high-quality health care, and we already pay enough health taxes to support that. High-quality healthcare costs less than the shoddy, mediocre care now delivered in the United States.
- We have inefficient, mediocre health care in the United States because that is what generates the highest profits for healthcare corporations. Prior to the COVID-19 pandemic, our national debt was historically due to the corporate welfare we taxpayers have been forced to give to the medical-industrial complex. Who forces us to make this gift? Politicians from both major political parties. There is not a dime's worth of difference between the parties when it comes to the essential features of health policy proposed by each.

Here's an idea. Tell your Congressional candidates you will not vote for them unless they promise to get the federal government out of the way so that states can attempt real, sustainable health-system reform. Call them, text them, email them, flood their campaign offices with demands that they publicly commit to support federal legislation that enables real, sustainable health-system reform at the state level, with federal oversight. Just watch how fast these politicians change their tune on health care after the first politician loses office because he/she fails to stop wasting tax dollars on healthcare corporate welfare.

In our absurd angst about socialism, we Americans are failing to capture the already massive magnitude of federal government involvement in our health care. In addition to the 122 million citizens on Medicare, Medicaid, and military health plans, there are millions more on CHIP, state and local government employee plans, and federal employee plans. Add to that the additional millions who receive VA health care and

Obamacare subsidies, and the total approaches 200 million Americans with some form of direct government health care. Further, remember that private-employer health plans exist because of a massive federal tax credit that has propped them up since World War II. No wonder most of the money flowing (over $4 trillion/year) into the United States' healthcare delivery is from taxes. As mentioned, Americans pay the world's highest healthcare tax burden. Without public monies, there would be no American health care.

This is the healthcare system we have chosen for the past seventy-five years; it is not socialism. We need to stop pretending we can now somehow choose to have health care without government involvement.

"Positive externality" refers to a situation when someone other than the buyer or seller in a market has a legitimate interest in the outcome of a transaction. One example of this is when the general public has an interest in assuring the best care for a patient with a communicable disease. We have massive infusions of tax dollars into health systems because of positive externalities.

Finally, the inverse relationship between price and demand does not hold for health services. No one ever bought an appendectomy because it was on sale. And, as mentioned in chapter 2, no diabetic willingly forgoes insulin even if the price skyrockets. Demand for health services is determined by epidemiology (which is the science studying how often disease and injury happen), not price. Health care is not a market commodity.

Congress has abysmally failed us on health care. Hyperpartisanship is part of the problem, but the massive campaign donations and lobbying power of the medical-industrial complex assure that both parties defend business as usual in healthcare delivery. Cost is our principal healthcare problem. The federal debt is burgeoning with pandemic-related spending, but it will continue to grow into the future because of unfunded healthcare costs. The health-insurance business model is incredibly ineffi-cient (wasting up to $500 billion per year), and health care in the United States is poor in quality (wasting up to $700 billion per year). We don't need more money in American health care; we need to reduce the inefficiency and quality waste inherent in healthcare business as usual.

I don't think Congress will ever pass Medicare for All, the progressive version of national health-system reform. President Biden has repeatedly said he would veto any bill that guaranteed universal health care to all Americans at a federal level. But Congress should be able to agree to allow states to attempt sustainable health-system reform. In the past, a number of Democrats have co-sponsored bills, such as the State-Based Universal Health Care Act (H.R. 3775 in the current congres-sional session), that would strengthen the power of states to reform healthcare systems and even allow neighboring states to band together to achieve better regional healthcare delivery. Obamacare itself anticipates that states will play an increasingly prominent role in reforming healthcare delivery. I believe many Republicans (or former Republicans like me) would agree that state-based health-system reform is a logical step in our constitu-tional form of government.

I urge all voters during the coming election cycle to carefully inquire of their congressional candidates whether they will seek enactment of the State-Based Universal Health Care Act or something akin to it.

4

RUNNING THROUGH THE
POLITICAL ICEBOX

Congress is currently gridlocked by two parties vying for dominance as an end in itself, with no real intent to help all Americans receive the gift of health care we have so generously funded through taxation. Rarely does anything actually get done. As a nation, we are limited by this political morass; our highest aspirations are never realized. We can't seem to do big things as a nation anymore. It is as if Congress has a perpetual wish that the nation will self-destruct. Therefore, I do not foresee a day when Congress will actually act to sustainably reform our healthcare system. Instead, I imagine an American healthcare system that is state-based (with oversight from the federal government) and nonprofit, delivering better private-sector care that is simply and publicly financed. Such a system must guarantee medically necessary care for every resident in the United States of America without requiring point-of-service payments.

I dare to propose healthcare reform based on the original conservative principles I was taught while growing up in suburban Arizona in the 1950s and 1960s. Like Goldwater trying to balance states' rights with civil rights, I recognize the inherent potential contradictions of original conservatism. But fear of health-system reform leading to public funding for privately delivered health care based on the often-articulated possibilities of loss of freedom and violation of markets leading to socialism is neither factual nor reasonable. It is merely the money power of the medical-industrial complex endeavoring to prolong its reign by working upon the prejudices of the people.

State-based health-system reform with regionally cooperative private-sector healthcare delivery and unified public, simple financing is the only conservative way forward for American health policy. It is simultaneously fiscally, morally, and constitutionally conservative.

I often spend a couple of hours at a time in City Creek Canyon. It's an ideal place for jogging, and it was especially ideal during the COVID-19 pandemic, when it was nice to be outdoors and windblown.

The paved road that meanders through the canyon is a gradual ascent from the Salt Lake Valley floor (at 4,200 feet above sea level) to the picnic pavilions five and a half miles up (at 6,600 feet above sea level). Though I've completed the eleven-mile round trip many times, mostly I turn back at the four-mile mark. In winter, though, the snowplow employed to keep the road open to the water-treatment plant stops just short of the three-and-a-half-mile mark, so my winter runs are generally shorter than at other times during the year.

As I jog, I traverse open meadows and pass through the shadows of deciduous and evergreen trees, the denizens of the riparian canyon bottom. Deer and squirrels are plentiful, and I have encountered the resident fifty-member wild turkey rampart on numerous occasions. I've also seen moose, elk, fox, coyotes, bobcats, and cougars. Recently, a fellow runner warned me that he had seen a wolf in the canyon (which seems unlikely to me).

City Creek Canyon is a gift the citizens of Salt Lake City give to themselves. Every time I jog through it, I try to remember to pray thankfully for the many blessings that have enriched my life. This canyon is where I offered a prayerful thanks for my rescue by the Davis County Sheriff's Department helicopter. It's where I pray for the help I need to turn the gratitude I feel for my many blessings into actions that matter in the lives of my brothers and sisters in the family of God. I have probably run more than twenty thousand miles in the canyon during the past twenty years, so I've had time for many prayers and much contemplation.

At about the one-mile mark, there's a bend in the canyon road where an uphill runner turns from heading generally north to an easterly direction as the road, which follows the creek bed, curves around a substantial, steep mountainside. That mountain is tall enough to completely block the sun from shining on the canyon bottom during the winter months when it is tracking its course in the southern sky.

In winter, then, just after rounding that curve and passing the one-mile marker, I jog into a stretch of road that is shaded and therefore icy and frigid. It's what we City Creek Canyon runners call the "Icebox." It's where the sun doesn't shine in the winter. It's why I dress warmly when winter jogging, and it's why I press forward with extra effort so I can reach the light and warmth of the sun on the other side. Every time I run through the Icebox in winter, it reminds me of the death wish Congress seems to have for the nation, and I wonder how we can get through this toxic political mess and regain our national will to do big things.

This mix of self-destructive political behavior seems to cry out for an institutional rescue of the American people, and it reminds me of two difficult City Creek Canyon experiences. The first is the previously recounted hike that required a helicopter rescue. The other is an earlier hike I managed to finish without calling for help, though I was physically in worse shape and the canyon itself was gravely threatened.

On the morning of July 29, 2008, my daughter-in-law

dropped her husband, my son Andrew, and me off at the gated entrance to City Creek Canyon. We had planned to hike the length of the paved road on that hot summer day and then ascend a steep, two-mile trail to a 7,500-foot elevation rim between our canyon and its neighbor to the south, Red Butte Canyon. From there we would scramble over the top of Little Black Mountain and down its western face into my neighborhood and return to home.

Even though it was a fifteen-mile trip, Andrew and I believed it was easily doable, even with the arduous climb to the rim. Granola bars and water in hand, we set off.

The first six miles were readily accomplished on five-plus miles of paved road followed by less than a mile of easy trail. As we started up the steep rim trail at midday, the temperature already exceeded ninety degrees Fahrenheit. Though we were shaded by the abundant forty-foot pines on the north slope of the rim between the canyons, the heat and the climb pushed us to heavy perspiring.

We reached the rim and, while looking down into Red Butte Canyon, finished off our water and granola bars. As we emerged from the pines and scrambled over the rocky top of Little Black Mountain, we could see a column of smoke coming from City Creek Canyon. Once at the top with a clear view all the way to the Great Salt Lake in the west, we could see that the smoke came from a wildfire about two miles above the entrance to the canyon on its north wall. With not a cloud in the sky, there could have been no natural explanation for the fire; it had to be human caused.

Andrew and I had spent much of our energy on the surprisingly difficult scramble over the top, and we were dehydrated. As we began the steep descent, the going became increasingly difficult. Our pace slowed to a crawl as we picked our way past slick, gravelly trail sections, barely avoiding a fall.

Meanwhile, the fire across the canyon picked up in intensity and rapidly spread concentrically from its point of origin. Fixed-wing aircraft began dropping red plumes of fire retardant around the edges of the blaze; ground-based crews couldn't reach the fire. It occurred to me that we were so exhausted we would not be able to escape the flames if the fire crossed the canyon and climbed its south wall toward us.

Coming off the steep upper descent onto the final four miles of more gradually sloped trail, I was noticeably dragging, not able to even ride gravity into a reasonable stride. By now, the fire had burned 150 acres. The fixed-wing aircraft had been replaced by a tag team of helicopters dumping bucketloads of water on the hotter spots. With one eye on the fire, I told Andrew to go on ahead of me, get home, replenish himself, and wait an hour before coming back to help me if I had not yet arrived. With that, he left.

I trudged on alone, unable to muster much more than a stumble downhill. When I was too weak to stand, I found a rock to sit on for a few minutes. I made agonizingly slow progress thereafter, but the fire seemed under control, thanks to government-organized aerial firefighting. It eventually burned a total of 180 acres, but I arrived home safely just before Andrew started back uphill to find me.

In City Creek Canyon, I have lived through long, exhausting hikes for which I was poorly prepared. I've needed rescue, and I've gotten it. I am grateful for those government services. I have seen massive flooding bring out the best volunteer efforts from average Utahns. Government services extinguished the wildfire in City Creek Canyon that, left unchecked, could have consumed me and invaded neighboring communities. We Americans, when playing our best governance game, can work wonders. I know. I have been the beneficiary.

But we are underperforming as a nation. We can no longer have nice things, it seems. We can't seem to dream big and get things done. We are a weak and exhausted nation, sitting on a rock in the wilderness, dehydrated and worn down by the heat of our endless arguments with each other. It's like we are continually jogging through an icebox where the sun doesn't shine in the winter of our endless ire, freezing us out from the goodness inherent in our nature and the opportunities offered by our natural resources.

A wildfire burns in our democratic republic, and our political parties use the fear and flames to stampede us into settling for false dichotomies instead of well-thought-out policy, indolent incumbents instead of the fresh energy and ideas of newcomers, and the sinister influence of predatory wealth and religious factions instead of general welfare through constitutional process.

The term *socialism* is a case in point. The fake conservatives of today harass the electorate with endless monologues about the evils of "socialism," as if the nation were actually about to be overrun by Comrade Lenin himself. These monologues are devoid of real definitions or facts because this is demagoguery at its most sinister level.

Borrowing from the Cold War Era the fear of communist dictatorships that combined a version of state ownership of most enterprise with cruelty-based autocracy, today's anti-socialism rants insist that non-Republican candidates are bent on stealing America's wealth, guns, livelihood, homes, and families. Never mind that no major American candidate to my knowledge has ever advocated for state ownership of any industry.

"Socialized medicine" is a term frequently slung around as if it were a real option under discussion for imminent implementation. Again, I have never heard of any major candidate anywhere in the United States who has made that a plank of his or her platform. To be sure, there are publicly owned hospitals and publicly employed physicians and other health professionals in the United States who would fit the definition of socialized medicine. One example is the Veterans Administration. But nobody is advocating that all hospitals become public property and all physicians, nurses, dentists, physical therapists, and other medical practitioners become public employees. Socialized medicine is simply not on anyone's political wish list in the United States, and it never has been.

In fact, the only real socialism going on in American health care is not the public ownership of hospitals or physician practices but the public ownership of massive healthcare liabilities while healthcare assets are privatized for profiteering. It's called "lemon socialism," defined as a system wherein financial successes are credited to the private sector, while their failures are transferred to the taxpayers through bailouts. Anyone who has paid attention to our nation's financial woes recognizes how lemon socialism is a most apt description of the American economy.

It is also applicable to our healthcare system, though here it is better called "lemon-cherry socialism." healthcare costs for Americans will be more than $4 trillion this year, approaching 20 percent of our gross domestic product. Most of that—nearly 70 percent—is paid by taxation. Many years ago, health insurers did not want the responsibility of paying for the health problems of the poor and elderly—two groups of healthcare lemons—so they pushed those populations onto the taxpayers' shoulders.

However, health insurers realized that some of the beneficiaries of government programs are relatively healthy; the proper industry term here is *cherries*, as in "cherry-picking." So they lobbied successfully for the "business" opportunity to provide health financing to selected groups of these patients in Medicaid-managed care and Medicare Advantage plans. These plans actually cost the taxpayer more than traditional government programs because the private health-insurance business model is all about avoiding risk, not managing it. The plans inventively enroll healthier people and take their government subsidies while they are well and then push them back into traditional government programs when they become sick and need care. The private sector picks the cherries, and the public sector gets the lemons.

One elderly woman, recently widowed, was in need of replacing her deceased husband's retirement-based Medicare supplemental plan, including coverage for medications. Her daughter worked in physician's office and was therefore savvy about various Medicare policies and offerings. In the course of her employment, she had discovered that Medicare Advantage plans frequently did not pay enough for services rendered. In fact, the physician she worked with had made a determination that selected Medicare Advantage plans, including those offered by United Health Care, were simply unreasonably low in reimbursement, and the office staff was instructed to not accept those plans. On her mother's behalf, she began searching for a Medicare supplement plan, not a Medicare Advantage plan. Her inquiries produced a response from someone who identified herself as a Medicare plan "representative." Though the daughter intended to keep her mother from purchasing a Medicare Advantage plan, and though both mother and daughter were assured this "representative" was not selling such a plan, ultimately, when they took her mother for a medical appointment with the new plan, it became apparent that they had, in fact, been sold a United Health Care Medicare Advantage plan. Deceptive sales tactics are often how these plans do business. Once in Medicare Advantage, it is difficult, if not impossible, to actually change to a Medicare supplemental plan.

Bill Semple, board chair for the Colorado Foundation for Universal Health Care, describes well who has the "advantage" with Medicare Advantage plans:

> "The advantage in Medicare Advantage is return on investment. The advantage is for the shareholders in insurance companies, including the top executives, paid largely through stock options.

Medicare Advantage is designed for beneficiaries who don't need much health care, yet want to believe they will be covered in time of need. Even for the healthy, hearing, dental, and vision coverage is a plus. Not having to pay for a supplemental plan, as in traditional Medicare, is another.

Advantage plans are paid on a per member, per month basis, and this on a risk adjusted basis, attempting to adjust for those with greater needs. So the basic incentive is to cover the relatively healthy, while coding them as maximally sick to increase reimbursements, then driving away those with increasing medical needs. (A related incentive, when health care must be paid for, is to collude in paying excessive drug, hospital, and medical equipment charges, to create a powerful, price-fixing, legal cartel to reinforce the status quo).

Do people tend to choose the appeal of Advantage plans when first a beneficiary, then switch to traditional Medicare as more needs arise? Yes. Not advertised in Advantage plans are the deductibles that can be separate for drugs and other care, the narrow provider networks with the related surprise billings, the frequent requirements for prior authorizations, and sketchy claims denials. The out-of-pocket maximums exclusive to Advantage plans sound good until needed to be met year after year. Added to the insults is the reality that supplemental plans have fixed premiums only for the first six months of eligibility; if someone wants to switch from Advantage to traditional Medicare and purchase a supplemental, the premium may be multiples of the initial rate, or refused entirely.

Medicare Advantage is an advantage to the relatively wealthy few. For those who need health care, it is a con."[1]

American socialism, the kind we should *really* fear, is better known as *corporate welfare*, and it is at its finest in health care (as well as in Wall Street bailouts). We Americans tax ourselves enough to pay for all medically necessary, high-quality, efficiently financed care that should be delivered in the United States *without raising any further tax revenues*. But we fail to deliver medically necessary care to many Americans because of the corporate welfare we are giving to health insurers, hospitals, and other parts of the medical-industrial complex.

Health insurers are not the only ones who play this game. Mike Leavitt, former governor of Utah and secretary of Health and Human Services under President George W. Bush, is fond of telling the story of his attempt to change the way Medicare pays for durable medical equipment. While he was head of the Department of Health and Human Services, his staff organized a trial competitive-bidding process for expensive equipment needed by Medicare patients. During the trial, a savings of up to 46 percent was demonstrated. But the program was killed before it became standard policy when medical-equipment sellers used lobbying to induce their representatives in Congress to obstruct the department's attempt to reduce taxpayer costs.

Medicare Part D, the pharmacy benefit for seniors, is yet another example of lemon-cherry socialism. Congress directed the Centers for Medicare and Medicaid services to set up a pharmacy-benefit program for senior citizens and then asked the pharmaceutical firms how much they wanted to charge the taxpayers for the drugs. Americans pay far more for brand-name medications as do the citizens of other countries. It's a blatant example of corporate welfare.

Bill Moyer recently said:

"Over the last two decades, the current members of the Senate Finance Committee have collected nearly $50 million from the health sector. A long-term investment that's now paying off like a busted slot machine. . . . A century ago, muckraking journalists reported that large corporations and other wealthy interests virtually owned the Senate, using bribery, fraud and sometimes blackmail to get their way. Jokes were made about the Senator from Union Pacific or the Senator from Standard Oil."[2]

One of the muckraking journalists of a century ago, David Graham Phillips, wrote an article in 1906 titled, "The Treason of the Senate," in which he said, "Treason is a strong word, but not too strong, rather too weak, to characterize the situation in which the Senate is the eager, resourceful, indefatigable agent of interests as hostile to the American people as any invading army could be."[3]

We have witnessed round after round of corporate welfare from Congress masquerading as health reform. Neither political party is acting in the interest of patients and taxpayers; they are eagerly pouring lemon-cherry entitlements for corporate hogs at the public trough. In effect, our politicians have set our health system on fire, allowing our patients to be harmed by business as usual in American health care so that special interests can use their predatory wealth to reap windfall profits. Yet when these members of Congress appear before us as candidates for reelection, they insist we should not fear the wildfire in our healthcare system, and they scaremonger about "socialized medicine."

It's time for us to turn the volume down on these political diatribes and rethink what really matters in our politics. Let's push through the icebox in American politics by un-electing the politicians of both parties who have created and massively funded corporate welfare. Throw the incumbents out of office because they have already failed to help solve America's healthcare crisis. This is how we can run through America's current political icebox.

5

HEALTH CARE: THE SENTINEL
DOMESTIC ISSUE OF OUR TIME

I s it possible to be nonpartisan in approach to supporting
candidates and issues in today's nation? Can voters actually
change party support and candidate choice election by election?
Can we Americans enjoy freedom from the dominance of political parties in our governance? Can we demand that we elect
leaders not to rule but to serve (as suggested by President Dwight
D. Eisenhower) by refusing to elect (or reelect) politicians who fail
to use the middle of the road to solve our nation's problems? Is
there a better time to start changing our national approach to
politics than now?

Now is the time for change, and the answer to whether we the
people of the United States can become nonpartisan is an
emphatic *yes*.

We have current examples of how this can be done. The two
men who received the Republican presidential nomination in
2008 and 2012, John McCain and Mitt Romney, respectively,
have demonstrated their patriotism by supporting and doing
what they each thought was just, correct, and according to inde-

pendent principle, even when what they did was outside partisan expectation.

healthcare policy became the final signature moment of Senator John McCain's career. He opposed the Patient Protection and Affordable Care Act (Obamacare) when it was passed—both on the merits of the bill and because of the unilateral, hardline Democratic politics behind it. And though he ran for his final Senate reelection on a theme of repealing and replacing it, when the issue came to a vote in the United States Senate in 2017, McCain famously did not follow the Republican Party line.

Just about the time I was getting lost in City Creek Canyon and needing helicopter rescue, John McCain was receiving a diagnosis of terminal brain cancer in Arizona. Republicans, then holding a slim majority in the United States Senate, held back the vote on the so-called "skinny" repeal of Obamacare, which was, in essence, repeal with no replacement because it was thought that they might need McCain's vote to prevail. Two Republican senators, Lisa Murkowski (R-AK) and Susan Collins (R-ME), had already declared their intent to vote against the "skinny" reform measure, but with McCain presumably voting for it, a fifty-fifty tie could be realized, which would then be broken in favor of passage by Vice President Mike Pence. This was President Trump's first signature legislative moment, and healthcare legislation again seemed likely to pass on a partisan basis, reversing Obamacare four years after its implementation.

With the voting held open on the Senate floor, Senator McCain was personally lobbied by Mr. Pence and then took a call from President Trump in the cloakroom of the Senate. Despite those efforts, he returned to the floor of the Senate and voted against the bill, later stating:

> "Our health care insurance system is a mess. We all know it, those who support Obamacare and those who oppose it. Something

has to be done. We Republicans have looked for a way to end it and replace it with something else without paying a terrible political price. We haven't found it yet, and I'm not sure we will. All we've managed to do is make more popular a policy that wasn't very popular when we started trying to get rid of it. . . . We've tried to do this by coming up with a proposal behind closed doors in consultation with the administration, then springing it on skeptical members, trying to convince them it's better than nothing, asking us to swallow our doubts and force it past a unified opposition. I don't think that is going to work in the end. And it probably shouldn't. The Obama administration and congressional Democrats shouldn't have forced through Congress without any opposition [or] support a social and economic change as massive as Obamacare. And we shouldn't do the same with ours."[1]

Ultimately, John McCain voted on that occasion according to what he knew to be right despite the fact that his vote went against the grain of intense partisanship.

Mitt Romney was John McCain's most vigorous rival for the Republican presidential nomination in 2008. Ultimately, Romney waited his turn for the nomination, which he received in 2012. During his run for the presidency that year, Romney received McCain's endorsement.

Mitt Romney and John McCain did not serve together in the United States Senate. Senator McCain died during the summer of 2018 while Mr. Romney was engaged in his first campaign for the Senate from Utah. Mr. Romney attended John McCain's funeral, and on social media, he eulogized the deceased senator as a friend and a giant in the United States Senate who would be missed by the nation.

Like John McCain, Mitt Romney has never supported the Patient Protection and Affordable Care Act (Obamacare). Both men did express at different points in time an interest in altering the federal tax policy that gives a tax credit to employers to offset the cost of employee health benefits in order to allow individuals to claim a tax credit for funds spent purchasing personal health insurance. This arcane approach to our nation's healthcare costs, of course, falls far short of any serious approach to health-system reform.

While McCain's last great moment in the national spotlight was his vote against the partisan grain to deny Mr. Trump's effort to repeal Obamacare, arguably Romney's first moment on the national political stage was as governor of Massachusetts, when he signed legislation creating a state-based health-insurance mandate that became the template for Obamacare, which was passed four years later.

Neither McCain nor Romney has ever really seriously grappled with the massive quality and inefficiency problems requiring reform in American healthcare delivery, but both encountered healthcare reform as the inescapable sentinel domestic issue that it is in the United States. Neither a change in tax policy nor a vote up or down on mandating the purchase of health insurance is real or sustainable health-system reform. But it is not coincidental that neither McCain nor Romney could escape an encounter with healthcare policy. Let's face it. All Americans are prone to gnawing health insecurity; the issue is perennially high on voters' minds.

Until we Americans actually face up to the massive cost problems inherent in the way we do healthcare business and definitively change how we deliver care, we will face recurring crises in health care requiring recurring responses from our elected officials. And until these elected officials care more about actually solving health-system problems than about partisanship and the political donations of the medical-industrial complex, nothing good on health care will come from Congress. We must insist that members of Congress love our patients more than they hate the other party.

John McCain and Mitt Romney have both taken a small step

in that direction by going counter to the partisan pressure in, respectively, preserving and anticipating Obamacare. Their willingness to withstand withering crossfire from their own party as they bucked partisanship—not only in healthcare policy but in articulating the truth about Mr. Trump and his high crimes and misdemeanors—can be seen as the rearguard action of original American conservatism in the Republican Party.

We as a nation can enjoy much-needed change in our healthcare system only if we overcome the problems related to partisanship and focus instead on the *health of the people*. Doing so will free our nation to create meaningful, workable solutions that benefit all Americans.

6

METAPHOR AND HEALING

There is a gap between rural and urban/suburban Americans on everything from life span to education to poverty. That gap, I believe, is the origin of the destruction of our body politic. Ask yourself: What are the resources and services that all Americans, urban or rural, old or young, need? Can we share something that makes all of us feel like we have a stake in our country and its governance? By visiting "even the least" of our American brothers and sisters consistently in some meaningful ways, can we stitch together the social fabric that has become so frayed? What does the urban-rural gap indicate about the way we all think of our national problems, including health care?

I have heard a number of voices from rural America speak up recently about the loss of healthcare services in their communities. In the past decade, 176 rural hospitals have closed, with another 450 rural hospitals currently at risk for closure. These hospitals were likely built with federal funds appropriated under the Hill-Burton Act. In addition to bringing needed care and services into rural communities, these hospitals brought good jobs to parts of the United States that desperately needed work. Business as usual in this nation's health care does not adequately provide for the healthcare needs of rural citizens. In the face of vanishing health services, many rural communities have turned to for-profit business interests to save their small hospitals from financial disaster only to discover that the medical-industrial complex takes profits without giving back. For-profit management of rural healthcare facilities inevitably leaves rural areas in further healthcare debt.

What works marginally in urban healthcare delivery makes no sense in sparsely populated farm country or frontier ranch wilderness. The notion that huge corporate healthcare interests can improve healthcare quality and encourage lower prices by competing for healthcare business is nonsense in urban areas, but it is totally unconnected to the reality of rural healthcare delivery, where sole providers of care obviously can't compete with themselves.

And let's stop talking about "coverage" instead of "care." Health insurers don't want to "cover" rural America, where people are less able to pay insurance premiums and more likely to be sick or injured. Patients don't need "coverage" anyway; when people are sick or injured, they need care. I suggest we start with the assumption that people all over this nation, perhaps especially those living in rural America, know best what kind of healthcare arrangements are needed where they live. Let's stop trying to enact and fund whatever health policy comes out of the medical-industrial complex. We already have the most profitable healthcare system in the world and therefore the least patient-centered and most expensive healthcare delivery among all developed nations—and one that is the least oriented to rural America.

The need for health care is universal. People die prematurely when their injuries cannot be treated in a timely fashion and when they cannot afford to buy lifesaving medications. While people certainly need more than just health care to live optimally, if we could find a way to transform American healthcare delivery so that every American, rural or urban, poor or wealthy, old or young, received medically necessary care guaranteed, attention could be given to other essential aspects of modern life.

healthcare delivery is administratively wasteful and of mediocre quality everywhere in the United States, but it's often simply absent in rural communities. Changing how healthcare business is done in the United States will require finding a way to serve every American patient. Let's begin with listening to rural Americans. They can tell us how best to organize healthcare delivery in their communities. We must build a healthcare system that puts patients first, no matter where they become sick or injured. Urban Americans often vacation in rural settings or drive through them. We all have a stake in building first-class care *everywhere* across America, including all along the interstate highway from Utah to Pennsylvania, which I have often traveled when visiting children and grandchildren.

Arguably, it was poor health and consequently rising death rates among white, middle-aged, non-college-educated voters, many living in rural areas, that brought Donald Trump the relatively few votes he needed to win the presidential election in 2016. Trump's surprise victory came as United States life expectancy dropped for the first time in my lifetime due exclusively to a half million excess deaths among white Americans under the age of sixty-five, while death rates among black Americans and Hispanics improved. Several observers, among them Nobel laureate Angus Deaton, have noted that the increasing mortality figures among white, non-college-educated Americans can be attributed to drug and alcohol overdoses, which almost quadrupled; suicides, which increased by 60 percent; and deaths from chronic liver disease and cirrhosis, which rose by a third. These deaths have been labeled "deaths of despair." As Jeff Goldsmith sums it up:

"In plainer words, white Americans in mid-life are basically killing themselves, either directly or with destructive personal habits, and in sufficient numbers to affect overall life expectancy in the country. It is not challenging to link the despair of older voters to de-industrialization and the economic hammering many Americans took in the 2008 recession, and thus to Trump's surprise victory.

About half of American households aged over 55 have no retirement savings. As a direct result of the crash, millions of older Americans lost the home equity they were counting on as a retirement cushion in the wave of foreclosures and job losses. A remarkable 86 million American households have, effectively, no spendable assets, and their asset position has actually declined in the past seven years. How strategically crucial to these voters was Trump's unconventional (for a Republican, at least) promise not to cut Social Security or Medicare, since tens of millions of hard-pressed baby boomers will be completely dependent on these programs in their seventies and eighties. Trump would have lost the election if he had followed traditional Republican policy dogma and pledged to "reform" these two safety net programs."[1]

The COVID-19 pandemic wreaked havoc on the nation's ability to receive much-needed health care. During the three-month period from February to May 2020, 5.4 million laid-off workers became uninsured, a record increase in uninsured adults in United States history. It far eclipsed the previous highest increase of 3.9 million nonelderly Americans becoming uninsured during the Great Recession of 2008–2009.

A real health emergency occurred in 2020. President Trump repeatedly promised remarkable reform of American health care but ultimately delivered only a few executive orders late in his presidential campaign about protecting patients with preexisting conditions and promising a couple of hundred dollars to assist patients with purchasing pharmaceuticals, with no details and no follow-through.

I am not arguing that health-system reform alone, as important as it is, will answer the call of Jesus of Nazareth for us to visit "the least" of our brothers and sisters. Clearly, the health of Americans is not solely the product of healthcare delivery. Far from it. Life expectancy grew dramatically in the United States from 1900 to 2010, as it did throughout the industrialized world, and not mostly because of remarkable progress in clinical science. It has been estimated that half of the total mortality reduction for major American cities between 1900 and approximately 1940 can be attributed to the introduction of water filtration and chlorination. Better nutrition, higher-quality education, and reduced violence, among many societal interventions, increased well-being and reduced the risk of death at every age. Improvements in nutrition and rising real incomes created by government antipoverty programs such as the Food Stamp Program allowed many people to fight off diseases that would otherwise have resulted in death.

In fact, American medical care itself has become too narrowly focused for its own good. This can be seen in the failure of American clinical scientists to understand the metaphorical/philosophical underpinnings of their own enterprise. While the use of metaphor is an essential feature of medical science, one particular metaphor, the so-called "mechanistic metaphor," so predominates the practice of medicine that it has been misconstrued as a description of reality. And this mistaking of a metaphor for truth has created a paradox: medical science is both a recognized success and a source of distress. The metaphorical physician, one who acknowledges the metaphorical nature of medical science, is free to use metaphor instead of being used by it. Freedom of imagination and faith, and freedom from excessive objectivity are potential benefits of the appropriate use of metaphor. Physicians should focus more attention on the metaphorical nature of medical science.

Metaphor, known to most as a figure of speech in which an analogy is made between two unlike objects, is an oft-used tool in medicine. Patients and physicians alike find metaphorical language to be the aptest and most concise way to express those things that would otherwise be difficult to describe, such as "stabbing pain" or "vegetative signs." Metaphor is also used to obscure meaning, such as when two physicians discuss "mitotic processes" while in the presence of a potential cancer victim. The practice of medicine, however, is even more fundamentally metaphorical than this because medical science, while not usually understood as such, is actually an example of applied metaphor.[2] Naturally, those physicians possessing knowledge of the function of metaphor in medical practice, termed here "metaphorical physicians," are free to use metaphor appropriately; others, unaware of the metaphor, will be used by it.

To understand how science is metaphorical, the term *metaphor* must be redefined to include things more complex than figures of speech. This extended notion of metaphor is well described by Colin Turbayne in his book, *The Myth of Metaphor.* As he defines it, metaphor exists wherever someone uses one sort of object to describe something of an entirely different sort (such as plants and patients when speaking of "vegetative signs") while at the same time acknowledging the pretense of the analogy (so no one confuses patients with plants). Included in this category of extended metaphors are fables, parables, allegories, myth, and models.[3]

A metaphor in this extended sense can be an effective tool, helping its users organize and communicate useful ideas; it is a way of focusing one's attention on certain important aspects of an object under study to understand it better. In this sense, a metaphor is a screen or filter (note the metaphorical language) that suppresses some parts of reality while emphasizing others.

"The chess metaphor, for example, used to illustrate war, emphasizes the game-of-skill features while it suppresses the grimmer ones."[4]

But Turbayne adds an important caveat to the use of metaphor:

> "One condition of the use of metaphor is awareness. More accurately speaking, this means more awareness, for we can never become wholly aware. We cannot say what reality is, only what it seems like to us, imprisoned in Plato's cave, because we cannot get outside to look. The consequence is that we never know exactly what the facts are. We are always victims of adding some interpretation. We cannot help but allocate, sort, or bundle the facts in some way or another."[5]

Metaphors are the way we interpret the world around us because we do not really know what the world is like. If the metaphorical nature of our interpretation is forgotten, we are at risk of blinding ourselves to our own tools. As Turbayne adds, "There is a difference between using a metaphor and being used by it, between using a model and mistaking the model for the thing modeled. The one is to make believe that something is the case; [the] other is to believe it." Forgetting the pretense in a metaphor changes the filter to a disguise, permanently suppressing some parts of reality.[6]

It may be a surprise to some that science, just as with other human endeavors, is actually based on a form of extended metaphor. The features of the predominant model, which can be referred to as the mechanistic metaphor, provide us with a case study of the potential for both good and bad found in every such analogy.

The creation of this metaphor is variously ascribed to Newton or Descartes or both. The dominant analogy of this metaphor can be found in the following quote from Descartes: "I have hitherto described this earth, and generally the whole visible world, as if it were merely a machine in which there was nothing at all to consider except the shapes and motions of its parts."[7] The medical corollary is that the study of the human body is like the study of a machine; the whole can be understood by reduction into parts (and subparts). The power of this metaphor is evident in the amazing accomplishments of modern-day medicine; everything from virgin births to mechanized body parts is now available, with more to come, seemingly ad infinitum.

The incredible success of the pronounced emphasis on the mechanistic metaphor in medical circles has encouraged some of its adherents to predict an eventual medical victory over death.[8] Medical scientists feel that as all the parts of the human machine are finally laid bare to scrutiny, the various causes of their malfunction will also be obvious. Thereafter, the search can be directed at finding an appropriate intervention point in the cause-effect illness sequence. Theoretically, all illnesses can be modeled on this mechanistic metaphor, and there, as Susan Sonntag notes in *Illness as Metaphor*, "Medicine's central premise is that all diseases can be cured."[9]

The faithful application of the mechanistic model to medicine over many decades, however, has not produced the universal health and happiness it seemed to predict. In fact, Dr. F. J. Ingelfinger has pointed out that 80 percent of all patients presenting to a doctor have self-limited disorders or conditions not improvable by medical intervention. Another approximately 10 percent of cases can be positively influenced by appropriate medicine. Unfortunately, however, Dr. Ingelfinger's figures indicate that most of the remaining 10 percent have iatrogenic [caused by a doctor or medical procedure] disease, leaving the "balance of accounts . . . marginally on the positive side of zero."[10]

Additionally, Dubos has challenged the idea that medical science was responsible for the improvement of general health in

the first half of the twentieth century, offering instead the explanation that public-health measures such as sewage control, water
treatment, and increased food quality and quantity were more
significant.[11] The amazing accomplishments of the mechanistic
model may not be improving the health of the general
population.

Medical science has also been criticized for things other than
its questionable impact on improving health. Authors such as
Ivan Illych, Susan Sonntag, Norman Cousins, Michael Crichton,
Martha Lear, and Lewis Thomas, among many others, have
made important comments about a wide range of medically
related topics, including philosophy, sociology, economics, and
history. All agree that traditional medical care, oriented as it is
toward Newtonian/Cartesian models, does not adequately deal
with human health issues.

There exists, therefore, a paradox. While the mechanistic
model has been shown to be useful, it is receiving increasing criti-
cism. Indeed, the problems surrounding the practice of medicine
seem numerous at present—among them rising healthcare costs,
more frequent malpractice and antitrust litigation, physician and
nurse burnout, and (perhaps consequentially) the undersupply of
doctors and nurses. Physicians are frustrated by these apparent
crises because they jeopardize the continued growth of both clinical science and the business models that spring therefrom. If
medical technology is to survive its own success, this paradoxical
treatment of the mechanistic model of medicine must be
resolved, and the inappropriate use of metaphor is at the center
of the controversy.

The metaphor itself is not wrong; it remains a successful
model for many problems. The reason for the many apparent
failures of the mechanistic metaphor is that we have violated the
rules of metaphor use: we have confused our model with reality.
Today's practitioner of medicine has never been made aware of
the metaphorical basis of medical science. It appears that physi-

cians are so impressed with the power of mechanistic thinking that they no longer differentiate between the model and reality. Medical scientists talk about knowledge and truth in biological medicine as if they actually possessed them. Where obvious gaps in biomedical "knowledge" appear, requiring overt use of metaphorical language to explain natural phenomena, medical scientists are often apologetic. An example is found in *Clinical Neuropsychology*: "We are too far from understanding brain-behavior relationships to be able to state hypotheses entirely without the use of metaphorical terms. Metaphor is not to be taken literally. Diagrams for example, may be used in a metaphorical way to present a hypothesis."[12]

Absent from this apology is the notion that all science is stated in metaphorical terms. Never does anyone write in a journal or stand in front of a class of medical students and proclaim, "What we are talking about is all pretense. Human beings in many ways are not at all like machines." Instead, medical students are required to learn the "facts" of physiology and other hard sciences as if those things were proven and hard and untouched by metaphor, and much is said about the need for more objective, double-blind, controlled, reproducible "facts" that confirm the power of mechanistic medicine. Those who are admired are those who provide more "scientific" evidence that the world is a machine. The supposed scientific ideal is to know about the world, not to believe in or feel strongly about things like metaphors. We are being used by our basic metaphor because, successful as it is, we have become certain that it is the truth.

Such certainty is unrealistic, however. Uncertainty creeps into Plato's cave on all sides. Human observation of natural events alters the nature of the subject, making the observation partially invalid, a phenomenon known as the observer effect. In medicine, the relationship between the observing medical doctor and the subject or patient is called *transference* or *countertransference*; each person has an effect on the other, making complete, objective characterization of the patient by another person, impossible. When partially invalid observations are used to form theories about nature, errors are bound to be made. Dr. Karl Rogers wrote:

"A slight error in a theory may make little difference in providing an explanation of the observed facts out of which the theory grew. But when the theory is projected to explain more remote phenomena, the error may be magnified, and the inferences from the theory may be completely false."[13]

In medicine, certain observations, though partially invalid, seem to confirm the mechanistic metaphor. For instance, the human heart is in many respects simply a mechanical pump, moving a liquid, blood, throughout an entire system, the extremities and organs of the human body. Other human phenomena, remote from these initial observations, may not fit the metaphor at all. Doctors and patients, however, being unaware of the metaphorical basis of medicine, continually attempt to explain all human problems in mechanistic terms, unknowingly increasing the likelihood of error.

Ironically, the overextension of the mechanistic metaphor into uncertainty is being pursued because of a human desire for more certainty. As pointed out in the book *Medical Choices, Medical Chances*:

"Certainty is an age-old dream. . . . Before the mechanistic age people sought comfort through ritual in the face of uncertainty. There were periods, for example, when people living at the mercy of uncontrollable natural forces gained a measure of psychological control by anthropomorphizing those forces and seeking to dominate them through the use of magic. Under the mechanistic paradigm people gained some real control over nature by acknowledging its separateness and learning how it worked. . . . It seemed as if the world were moving toward greater certainty.[14]

Under this illusion of certainty, patients continually approach doctors for answers to human problems. And in search of this certainty, doctors train for increasingly more years. A greater percentage of the total human effort, especially in the United States of America, is currently being placed into health care than ever before, with no real increase in the certainty of human health. It seems obvious, at least to me, that continued retreat to technological solutions is merely another form of comfort-seeking ritual. Business as usual in American health care merely exploits this human craving for certainty.

Because of its illusion of certainty, medicine has damaged our ability to deal humanely with uncertainty. Hayes has pointed out that while medical science has promised us immortality, it has actually "brought us closer to our own finitude and ultimate impotence. The modern physician is perhaps more face-to-face than his predecessors with the ultimate paradox of life, which is death, precisely because the awesome technology at his fingertips can only rearrange mortality, never avoid it."[15] Lewis Thomas, however, observed:

> We continue to share with our remotest ancestors the most tangled and evasive attitudes about death. . . . At the very center of the problem is the naked cold deadness of one's own self, the only reality in nature of which we can have absolute certainty, and it is unmentionable, unthinkable.We may be even less willing to face the issue at first hand than our predecessors because of a secret new hope that maybe it will go away. We like to think, hiding the thought, that with all the marvelous ways in which we seem now to lead nature around

by the nose, perhaps we can avoid the central problem if we just become, next year, say, a bit smarter.[16]

By our own insistence on mechanistic metaphors, we have denaturalized death by denying its necessity. What was once man's only certainty is now only a temporary failure, not something for serious consideration. Religious faith, once an important effort to dignify man's mortality, became indefensible in the face of the scientific striving for death-defeating facts. With the demise of overt faith now becoming so prevalent among all social strata, the language to explain human virtue, to arouse hope, and to decry evil has become dead vocabulary. In short, the strivings, vicissitudes, and values that would make our biographies human are of no interest to the purely scientific, for they are not mechanistic.

The mechanistic metaphor of medicine, therefore, has only limited application. When faced with the certainty of death, its technologies are powerless and sometimes harmful. It can force air into lungs, prevent polio, and remove inflamed organs, but it cannot assuage uncertainty, nor can it make life meaningful, for machines are certain and without meaning. These limits exist by the very nature of the metaphor and must be recognized, as must the metaphor itself, if attempts are to be made at improving on the past.

I remember caring for a patient in her late 60's while serving on the surgical service of a community hospital as a family practice resident. This woman had been hospitalized for 3 weeks before I became the resident responsible for her day-to-day care. A month before I met her, she had been a very healthy, active grandmother, who had experienced occasional discomfort on the right side of her abdomen. Worried that this symptom might be the harbinger of serious illness, and seeking the assurance (or certainty) that she was really not unwell, she presented her episodic complaint to a surgeon. The surgeon assumed, initially, that something was wrong with the patient's gall bladder, but his initial investigation with imaging studies did not confirm his clinical intuition. Rather than offer this healthy woman some reassurance that she was well and should tolerate the occasional discomfort, at least unless and until it became more severe, frequent, or in some other way definitive, the surgeon pursued more arcane clinical testing. Eventually his diagnostic pursuit was rewarded with a test result possibly indicative of an obstruction of the pancreatic duct. The surgeon offered the patient a surgery which he claimed could find and remove the obstruction.

The patient, now convinced that she was not healthy, opted to have the surgery. During the procedure, no obstruction was found. After the surgery, the patient was never well again. She began having nightly fevers. Eventually an abscess was discovered around her liver, which was next to the surgical field. Rather than take this patient back to the operating room and drain the abscess, the surgeon opted to treat her with antibiotics. As a result, the bacteria causing her abscess became resistant to many antibiotics. The fevers grew worse, her infection generalized throughout her body. She developed pneumonia, and then heart failure. She was intubated and sedated. Her kidneys failed. So she was placed on dialysis. Every failure of a body system induced the surgeon to order a mechanical substitute for the failure, but she did not improve, she worsened.

In a desperate attempt to reclaim the patient's health, the surgeon finally took her back to the operating room and drained the abscess. Immediately after the surgery, she seemed to be more stable. Her fever abated, her heart rate steadied, she required less oxygen, and her kidneys seemed to rally, lessening the frequency of dialysis. But she never woke up or responded to her family. She was being fed intravenously and was nutritionally losing ground. Every day my job was to check into all of the mechanical variables that are signals of body function and mechanically correct what seemed wrong: electrolytes, proteins, pH, vital signs, gas levels, etc. But the sum of these parts was no longer adding up to a functioning human being. She was obviously uncomfortable but unable to tell us what was wrong or respond in any meaningful way. She was slipping away from her family and medical care could not stop the slide.

Ultimately, an abscess reformed in her abdomen, sepsis reasserted its grip on her body, and she died, six weeks after being admitted to the hospital as a perfectly healthy person. The pursuit of certainty about her health had killed her one organ system failure at a time.

Doctors and patients alike must realize with Hayes that "the ability to live with paradox, uncertainty, finitude, and impotence and still find meaning in life is the sine qua non of the modern physician,"[17] or so it should be. Physicians who are informed about life only by collecting mechanical facts can never imagine the meaning of what is happening around them. The physician who practices with an awareness of the absolute limitations of the mechanical model must develop imaginative ways of dealing with the human problems existing outside the range of the mechanical. Such an effort will naturally address most of the major problems afflicting medical practice today. The metaphorical physician is free to use metaphor instead of being used by it. In a metaphorical society, the strivings, adversities, and values of each of us will bridge the gaps that keep us apart, such as the differences between urban and rural Americans, and we will find a way to serve every one of us.

7

THE METAPHORICAL PHYSICIAN

Perhaps the first freedom of metaphorical medical practice would be freedom from excessive objectivity. Enslavement to objectivity, rooted in the quest for certainty, has been a central cause for several of today's crises in medicine.

A patient in mechanistic medicine wants the certainty of a completely informed physician. Doctors respond by attempting to show that they know everything to secure the attention of their patients. In search of all the facts, the patient is typically subjected to multiple questions, extensive manual probing, phlebotomy, and radiation. Sometimes the patient is expected to produce various bodily fluids or secretions for further study. Occasionally, getting all the facts requires the patient to allow the invasion of several semipermanent needles or tubes or even subject himself to surgery. Consultants may be called in, and the medical literature is scanned.

The result, whether good or bad for the patient, is an outpouring of data sufficient to overwhelm even the most sophisticated, forcing the patient to assume that the medical effort has been complete. Doctors are rarely criticized for gathering too much data, but if they do not fulfill the expectations of fact-finding effort, they are scorned because a doctor of mechanistic medicine is rewarded for pretended objective omniscience.

Rising healthcare costs through increased reliance on technology as well as increased numbers of malpractice claims are natural associates of enslavement to such objectivity. Poor-quality care occurs not just through neglect but also through application of clinically inappropriate interventions even when well meant. These problems among physicians have their origin in medical education as students are principally rewarded for memorizing and developing a fund of objective knowledge. The pretense of objective omniscience is also partly responsible for medicine's trend to specialization; doctors feel less uncertain when they need pretend omniscience for only a restricted range of facts.

Freedom from excessive objectivity would change the nature of medical practice. No longer would patient care be exclusively an issue of applying double-blind, controlled, reproducible, tangible science because of the reality of nonmechanistic variables in every patient. These cannot be objectively known. The metaphorical physician is, therefore, not exclusively a fact-finder but also a problem-solver.

Doctors are useful to patients not because of what they know but because of wider experience in some types of human problems, whether that experience be from study or practice. Each human problem is a unique experience requiring unique solutions. Appropriate medicine must be responsive, not only to the specific disease itself, but to the patient's complicated mental and social being. Even well-practiced physicians will face unfamiliar problems as they move through their offices and hospitals. "No one in medicine," notes Binger, "is wise enough to comprehend what he daily beholds."[1]

Doctors must learn to develop strategies for dealing with the unknown without specializing or resorting to endless fact-finding or spectacular treatments. To this end, medical schools should reduce or eliminate lectures, multiple-choice exams, and rounds-manship that require memorized approaches to human problems; instead, they should encourage analytic and synthetic thinking among their students. Patients must also recognize the reality of nonbiological illness, for metaphorical physicians need patients who understand the function of metaphor in medicine. The patient will always be central to the solution of his or her own problems. Once a metaphorical approach to medical problems is adopted, the rewards for omniscience and objectivity will be replaced by premiums for problems solved. Says Binger, "All the sick man really wants is to get well by any method that works."[2]

As has been noted, the large margin of human life that cannot be scrutinized mechanically makes complete knowledge an impossible goal. Man will never have possession of enough facts to allow completely correct action in any sphere or activity. Each person can only believe that his or her experiences in some measure reflect reality and are therefore deserving of analysis. Inevitably, such analysis becomes an attempt to organize experience into a meaningful, understandable segment, such as a metaphor. If useful, such a metaphor will become a fixture in the individual's perspective on world events; he or she believes the natural world will usually match the expectations of his or her metaphors.

Belief in one's own experiences and thought processes is an essential part of the human makeup; to see is, in reality, to believe. Scientists, philosophers, clergymen, indeed, all men, must recognize that faith, not knowledge, is the basis for organized human progress. Faith in mechanistic science has made current technology possible, just as faith in God, when based on reasoned human experience, can make mortality more meaningful. Indeed, faith, or "the willing suspension of disbelief,"[3] is what energizes all good metaphors, whether they are created by

Newton, Shakespeare, or Jesus; man lives by faith in an endless variety of metaphors.

Another freedom of metaphorical medical practice, therefore, would be the freedom to have faith in more than one metaphor. For any one problem, different people will have differing solutions. Two different solutions may be equally helpful or disparately so, or they may complement each other, depending on the fit between the underlying metaphors and the presenting human situation. A person who has narrowed his personal spectrum of faith down to one or two metaphors will have a consequentially restricted problem-solving ability. Mechanists, for example, see words and other symbols as having only explicit meanings because all things must function as parts of the precise human machine. The word *disease* refers to a specific set of things, all of which result in biological changes. Where no such upset can be proved or presumed, no disease can exist, and no therapy need be undertaken. And if the biological change leading to disease is discovered, the mechanistic response is unrelenting medical therapy.

This is the thinking that resulted in our current crisis-oriented medical-care system, where prevention is underemphasized and death is institutionalized. The mechanistic metaphor is unnecessarily restrictive whenever it is the exclusive belief system for human health care. The metaphorical physician recognizes the usefulness of mechanistic medicine but also realizes that nonmechanistic illnesses afflict all people and require unmemorized, nonfactual metaphors for healing. Such metaphors make the patient's values, feelings, and prejudices an important part of the diagnostic process.

The avowed goal of the metaphorical physician is to optimize the well-being of the patient "by any method that works."[4] That might well mean not hospitalizing an ill patient when nonmechanical variables are more important than the biological aspect of disease. For instance, an elderly patient may feel that aggressive, hospital-based interventions which might prolong life are non-the-less unwanted. The patient's needs and desires are considered to be as important as the requirements of mechanistic medicine because no set of beliefs can dominate all others.

I once cared for an eighty-four-year-old woman with a history of schizophrenia. One of her delusions was that she had marble-sized dandruff flakes dropping from her hair that she would inhale while sleeping, thus suffocating her. She treated that dandruff problem by soaking her head in Lysol. Imagine the level of anxiety she lived with which could only be kept at bay by ritually sticking her scalp in a bucket of household cleaner. Despite her obvious mental limits, on one subject she spoke repeatedly and clearly, and that was that she did not want to die in a hospital. She had a comfortable home where she wished to remain until her demise, which she knew would be sooner rather than later.

So I had a dilemma one afternoon when called to the emergency room, where I found her being evaluated after a fall at home. There was no fracture, but the x-ray of her rib cage showed that she had pneumonia. I offered her inpatient IV antibiotic therapy for a few days with a promise that she would be discharged as soon as possible to finish her medication course with pills taken orally at home. She agreed to this believing I would follow through and discharge her as soon as possible.

Two and a half days later, at 4:00 a.m. on the morning I planned to discharge her, I received a call from her hospital nurse telling me she had a significant GI bleed that could rapidly cause her to lose enough blood that she would die. The on-call doctor caring for her in the hospital, who was not privy to the promise I had made, immediately started IV-fluid treatment followed by a blood transfusion. By the time I arrived to participate in the decision-making, a GI scope had found a source of hemorrhage in her stomach, and a surgeon had been consulted. My patient was unconscious and therefore unable to voice her opinion about what should be done. I did explain during the conference between the physicians and my patient's daughter, her only family, that the patient preferred to let nature take its course. But according to law, it was the daughter's decision, not mine, and she chose to have the surgeon go ahead and prep this woman for what he called "lifesaving" abdominal surgery. I stepped away from the situation and left it in the surgeon's care.

Late that same night, just before midnight, I received a phone call from the surgeon asking me to speak with the patient—who after treatment had awakened—and convince her to have the surgery. Apparently, she awoke as she was being wheeled into surgery, inquired where she was, and, upon discovering what had been planned, exclaimed, "Where is Dr. Jarvis? Why hasn't he kept his promise to let me go home?" She wouldn't sign the surgical consent form. I reminded the surgeon that she didn't want surgery. She bled out through her GI tract a few hours later and died in hospice. Mechanistic medicine was not the answer to this patient's needs.

The immediate effects of pursuing alternative healthcare options will be felt by those needing long-term care. Often, partially because of traditional medical practice, financial incentives keep patients institutionalized when they would be happier and better cared for elsewhere. Many chronic conditions respond better to nontraditional, outpatient therapies, such as those offered by Chinese medical doctors, than to western medicine. And much of the day-to-day management of health problems can be done by non-MD practitioners. The burden of health care can be shared with consequential beneficial cost savings and increased compliance. Thus, a metaphorical approach increases the number of viable healing options for the physician and the patient.

One final freedom resulting from metaphorical practice is the freedom to imagine. The human imagination is the most powerful tool available to us for dealing meaningfully with an uncertain, mortal world. It is that part of the central nervous system from which all metaphors come; it is what most distinguishes man from the rest of the animal kingdom. Because man can organize past experience into a new perspective on world events, future effort can be positively redirected; man alone among all species can willfully overcome instinct with intuition.

The immense power of the human imagination is demonstrated by the success of its creations, from flights into outer space to the best in fiction. However, the imagination fuels more than inventiveness; it also powers each individual human life with hope, inspiration, belief, and love. Imaginative living can also increase well-being, even under conditions of extreme disease, for "there is always a margin within which life can be lived with meaning and even with a certain measure of joy, despite illness."[5]

As the meaning and joy of life increase with imaginative efforts, a healthier state of being evolves. Indeed, there are connections between the imagination and the immune system. Kenneth Pelletier has reviewed the attempts of several researchers to understand the impact of the imagination upon healing. He writes, "Imagery has been demonstrated to be a sensitive reflection of a patient's emotional state as well as the means by which psychophysiological regulation is achieved."[6] Several essayists have also pointed out the importance of imagery in the human effort to make sense out of the commotion of the universe.[7] Though such imagery is still not within reach of the mechanistic metaphor (and may never be), the usefulness of a stimulated imagination for improving health seems sure.

The healing properties of the stimulated imagination are a by-product of its broader applications. When fully engaged, the imagination provides its owner with experiences that are quintessentially human: those most moving and penetrating. Whether sad, humorous, enraging, joyous, comforting, or stimulating, imaginative experiences are indelibly meaningful. The imagination, by tuning thoughts and feelings together, forms the individual's life experience into an orchestrated theme. That theme, whether played on piccolo or pianoforte, is that person's addition to the total human concert, and it earns either applause or embarrassed silence. Man's imaginative efforts are what dignify his existence, are what link him to his brothers and sisters. The imagination is what sharpens the "sense of participation in life."[8]

Traditional medical training, as has been previously noted, ignores the physician's imagination in an attempt to secure a large fund of biological knowledge. This discourages new physicians from attempting anything but standard diagnostic and therapeutic techniques with their patients that, though useful, are full of mechanistic error. Beyond limiting medical practices, however, the atrophied imaginations of many physicians effectively decrease their ability to cope well with the stress of healthcare delivery. The problems of physician drug abuse and suicide are reminiscent of what Albert Camus writes about the doctors involved in fighting the bubonic plague in his novel *The Plague*:

> "But the most dangerous effect of the exhaustion steadily gaining on all engaged in the fight against the epidemic did not consist in the relative indifference to outside events and the feelings of others, but in the slackness and supineness that they allowed to invade their personal lives. They developed a tendency to shirk every movement that didn't seem absolutely necessary or called for efforts that seemed too great to be worthwhile. Thus these men were led to break, oftener and oftener, the rules of hygiene they themselves had instituted, to omit some of the numerous disinfections they should have practiced, and sometimes to visit the homes of people suffering from pneumonic plague without taking steps to safeguard themselves against infection, because they had been notified only at the last moment and could not be bothered with returning to a sanitary service station. There lay the real

danger; for the energy they devoted to fighting the disease made them all the more liable to it."[9]

Physician burnout is partially due to a lack of creativity among doctors who have only mechanistic means of expression and are therefore cut off from their fellow human beings.

Likewise, patient burnout, the complication of physical disease by despair and hopelessness, is the result of patients ignoring the imaginative healing powers of their own minds. All patients must learn, with Norman Cousins, that they should "never . . . underestimate the capacity of the human mind and body to regenerate—even when the prospects seem most wretched."[10] A person with no imagination is already ill.

Freedom of imagination and faith and freedom from excessive objectivity are potential benefits of the appropriate use of metaphor. By forgetting its metaphorical origins, mechanistic medicine has raised expectations of itself that can never be fulfilled. The continued effort to extend the mechanistic metaphor has resulted in increased cost and specialization with limited return in improved health. Patients and doctors alike are disappointed in the result. What is needed now is recognition that medical science does not expose the truth about human beings; it only extends a useful metaphor. The existence of other metaphors useful for solving human problems is certain, and the multiple problems of medicine practiced today will not be solved until multiple metaphors are used more flexibly. A focus of discussion in medicine today should be on metaphor. It is long overdue for physicians to broaden their approach to problem-solving for their patients.

As an example of the power of expanding metaphorical approaches to solving patient problems, I offer my experience assisting patients with addiction problems as a primary-care physician alongside my experience as a lay pastoral leader (bishop) in a congregation (ward) of The Church of Jesus Christ of Latter-day Saints, counseling parishioners with addiction and their families. As a family doctor, my training helped me identify people with substance abuse problems, often before they were ready to ask for my help. I knew the mechanics of how drugs and alcohol affected various organ systems and could draw blood and conduct other diagnostic evaluations that supported a diagnosis of substance abuse. Incidental findings on studies done for reasons unrelated to drug and alcohol consumption could provide me with clues about whether a patient might be drinking too much, for instance. But these mechanical facts were never enough to help the patient address the problem of addiction.

Part of the reason for the reluctance of people to be forthcoming about drug and alcohol problems is, of course, the stigma of criminality attached to the issue. If addiction had historically been considered a disease in the United States, as it is, for instance, in Portugal, people would generally be less likely to hide the problem from their doctors. As noted in an opinion piece published in the *New York Times*, "It is impossible to treat addiction as a disease and a crime simultaneously."[11] That switch, from characterizing addiction as a crime to considering it to be a disease needing treatment, is a metaphorical switch in and of itself.

However, as a lay minister, I found addiction problems required another kind of approach. Most of the addicts I counseled as a bishop understood everything there was to know about their drug or alcohol habits from the perspective of both crime and disease. Many had already served time or were doing so when I met them. All knew about the medical requirements for detoxification from the drug of choice and about the pharmacological properties of the medications used to assist them in avoiding relapse once they chose to undergo rehabilitation. They were not seeking my help mostly for either legal or medical problems, though those issues did come up often.

Rather, my parishioners with addiction problems had trouble

with spiritual issues. Shame, for instance, far more than the stigma of a criminal record, haunted their thoughts and led them to belittle themselves and essentially give up on any meaningful future. Whatever dreams they might have had as children had been shredded by their recurring failures to master their weakness for abusing a chemical substance. Experience in addiction made them doubt anything and everything about themselves. In frustration, many told me they had given up their belief in God, but as we talked, it became apparent that what they were really thinking was that God could never care for someone like them and, therefore, out of shame, they would abandon their faith.

Lack of faith in God caused by having no hope for oneself had a significant consequence for these people, many of whom had been at one time, by nature, kind and thoughtful people. Because of self-imposed shame, a feeling of worthlessness in one's own and, by extension, God's eyes, they came to believe they had nothing to offer anyone else. Feeling useless to society, to one's family, or to anyone makes one begin to withdraw from meaningful human contact, become unkind, and ultimately dishonest with others. These tendencies wreak havoc on families, and they became the leading reason these people came into my office.

In my spiritual capacity, I was given the resources to assist these families through invoking any or all of these metaphorical approaches to addiction, individually or simultaneously. I could offer to arrange detox or rehab care, with financial backing of church resources if needed. I could feed and house someone temporarily, giving the family time to sort through the hurt feelings and ruined relationships shame causes, and even give the family permission to exclude an addict indefinitely if that was what they needed, knowing I could be a caring backstop for their loved one. As a minister, I was allowed to go to court and into jail to be with and assist those ready to address the sanctions of society for their behavior. And when they were ready to rejoin society, I could help them find jobs and start new lives. I did all of these things at various times during my service as bishop.

The key for me was discovering that addiction is not limited to mechanical, physiological findings, nor is it only a problem of breaking the law. It is also not just about the spiritual problems of shaming oneself so much that there can be no faith in God or hope in oneself, and therefore no interest in or charity for others. These various ways of addressing addiction are examples of metaphorical approaches to human problems. Each has a value, and each may need to be invoked, or not, to best solve the problems a particular individual has. We need a healthcare system that can be a place for that kind of imaginative problem-solving.

8

THE HOW OF PROGRESS AND
CONSERVATIVE HEALTH REFORM

The simultaneous need for substantial healthcare reform and critical political change at the present moment in the United States is not mere coincidence. We Americans allowed a remarkably bad health-financing business model to take root in our country through a political decision made seventy-five years ago when bipartisanship was much more common. While we were publicly funding a massive increase in medical education, facilities, and research during the second half of the twentieth century, we also increasingly allowed the suppliers of private health financing and medical goods and services to amass megafortunes they used to protect their windfalls, profiteering through massive lobbying and campaign support on a bipartisan basis.

The increasing dependence of both parties on medical-industrial-complex money hollowed out any original intentions to help patients, leaving only the drive for dollars as the business model of American healthcare delivery. Even the efforts to fund health care for the poor, the elderly, and children—Medicaid, Medicare, and CHIP—which originally seemed to be idealistic bipartisan efforts, have been rechanneled into avaricious business enter-prises—lemon-cherry socialism at its worst. While poor-quality health care is not the only way American government is failing its people, its delivery cuts at the very heart of modern living. The poor health of America's middle class has embittered them to the point that they are abandoning any pretense of supporting the great American experiment in self-governance. Mr. Trump's will-ingness to slash and burn the entire democratic process, including major institutions of government, was a selling point for voters for whom those institutions no longer held any promise.

Though health-system reform will be only a part of the polit-ical lift needed to bring the American electorate back into align-ment with original constitutional principles, I believe that doing something sustainable about health care is a necessary first step because of the enormous cost of business as usual in American health care.

The American economy, as big as it is, cannot continue to sustain annual increases in the percentage spent on health care for the simple reason that as the proportion of gross domestic product spent on health care rises, there is a consequent decrease in spending on all the other domestic products and services that must be purchased in order to make possible optimum health and the pursuit of life, liberty, and happiness.

The uniquely bad way Americans finance health care—private for-profit health insurance—makes massive increases in health spending inevitable. People think that health insurers make money by reducing how much is spent on health care, but that is not really true. Yes, health insurers reduce what they actu-ally pay for health care by deploying legions of bureaucrats to enforce benefit denial and invoke the related business practice of excluding people likely to need health care from acquiring health insurance in the first place. But in addition to that, insurers make very accurate predictions about the forthcoming healthcare costs they will pay and then simply run up the premiums, deductibles, copayments, and coinsurance to cover those costs plus 20 percent or more overhead. High costs mean higher actual overhead percentages and therefore higher profits. The "market" for healthcare services is not bearing these high costs because, actually, the American economy, and therefore the American way of life, is crumbling underneath them. No wonder economists have long predicted that the United States must corral health expenditures lest they engulf so much of the gross domestic product that the wheels fall off of our economy.

These facts have many progressives loudly calling for a national single-payer system through expanding Medicare to fund health care for all Americans. I credit Senator Bernie Sanders for serving as the voice that finally broke through to national audiences about the broad virtues of single-payer health-system financing.

Federal solutions, like Medicare for all, are what the progressive community commonly reaches for, and it is what Senator Sanders is proposing. But original American conservativism favors reserving to the states those policy arenas not explicitly granted by the Constitution to the national government, such as health-system policy and reform. This is a debate we should be seeing between progressives and conservatives. One would think, therefore, that conservative politicians would be proposing legislation that allows states optimum latitude in fashioning health policy, including establishing a state-based single-payer system in one or more states. This is what Senator Mike Lee promised he would do when he first ran for the United States Senate in 2010. But that was an empty promise, and the faux conservatives of today's Republican Party have nothing constructive at all to say about real, sustainable health-system reform, not even at the state level. As Goldwater indicated, American conservatism is finished when it has nothing useful to say about the proper place of state governments in our constitutional array of governance.

There are, however, a few progressive members of Congress

who can see the value of expanding the options for health-system reform among the various state governments. They can see that the politics of health-system reform forbid a federal single payer ever even receiving a congressional hearing, much less passing through a filibuster in the U.S. Senate. The current president of the United States has loudly declared that he will veto any federal single-payer bill that makes it to his desk.

Therefore, beginning with Representative Jim McDermott (D-WA) more than a dozen years ago, a couple dozen progressive members of the House of Representatives have introduced into each session of Congress the federal legislation needed to make state-based single-payer health-system reform possible. Representative McDermott, a psychiatrist by professional training and experience, entitled his state-based health-reform bill, "The States' Right to Innovate in Health Care Act." The current version of this legislation, principally sponsored by Representative Ro Khanna (D-CA), is entitled, "The State Based Universal Health Care Act," and it has the following purpose: "to establish a flexible framework under which States can provide comprehensive universal health coverage to all of their residents."

Reporting on this proposed legislation in 2019 when Representative Khanna first introduced it into the most recent previous Congressional session, Sarah Kliff of the *New York Times* wrote on November 8, 2019, in an article entitled, "What if the Road to Single-payer Led Through the States?":

"Federal rules can make it difficult for states to create single payer systems. Medicare, for example, accounts for 20% of national health spending and covers 60 million people. The federal government has full control of the program, deciding what it covers and how it pays doctors and hospitals. The federal government also regulates a large share of private health plans, typically those provided to workers at large companies, under a set of rules known as ERISA (the

Employee Retirement Income Security Act, passed in 1976). This means that states that want to introduce a single payer plan would have to leave (out) enrollees in those plans, as well as those using Medicare plans. . . . The Khanna legislation would try to get rid of those hurdles. It envisions a waiver that would allow states to take over the Medicare money that flows their way and combine it with funding for Medicaid, the Affordable Care Act marketplaces, the Tricare program that covers military families and funds for veterans' health care. A state would need to submit a plan for how it would use those funds to cover at least 95% of its population within five years, then cover the remaining uninsured within a decade."

The Khanna legislation would make it possible for the various states to choose to consolidate health financing and policy-making and organize an effort to simplify the administration of health benefits and improve the quality of care delivered in the state. This is much like the history of provincial health-system reform during the 1970s in Canada after Saskatchewan became the first province to enact single-payer health financing after World War II. In the United States, Medicaid, a shared federal/state program providing health financing to the poorest citizens in the country, was enacted in 1966 with only half of the states initially opting to participate. By 1982, when Arizona organized its Medicaid program, all fifty states offered the program. Each state learns from the others, providing a fulfillment of the oft-cited observation that the states are the laboratories of democracy in the United States.[1]

Beyond the advantages of staying within the framework of American constitutional governance, state-based health-system reform characterized by better quality private-sector care and unified, simplified public-sector financing has the potential to optimize the delivery of care within each of the fifty states, each with its unique needs and parameters. Utah, for instance, has relatively low per capita healthcare costs and a population concentrated along the Wasatch Front—a two-hundred-mile stretch in Northern Utah with Salt Lake City in the middle. A remarkably full range of healthcare services is available at the sophisticated medical centers in Salt Lake City, which draw patients from surrounding intermountain states, including parts of Wyoming, Idaho, Montana, Nevada, and Colorado. Because of this regional dependence on the specialty care located in Salt Lake City, it is easy to forecast that if the states were allowed to enact substantial health-policy changes, a multi-state health system could emerge in the intermountain west.

The remainder of Utah, spreading south of the Wasatch Front area, is sparsely populated but rich in attractions, with five very popular national parks, seven national monuments, four national forests, and many other popular landmarks and recreational areas. These attractions draw millions of visitors to Utah each year, principally in the warm weather months. Utah's smaller cities and towns, which are home to smaller medical facilities, are where recreational injuries are often initially treated.

The health-system profile of Utah is completely different from the health services needed in an eastern state like Massachusetts, which has a very high per-capita healthcare cost and a relatively high population density, even away from the Boston metro area. A health policy developed in Washington, DC, would not likely optimally serve either Utah or Massachusetts.

Pursuing the passage of the State Based Universal Health Care Act is how original American conservatives can, as Goldwater said, "demonstrate and communicate the difference between being concerned with the sick [who are] without medical care and believing that the federal government is the proper agent for" solving this problem. Joining progressive supporters, such as Representative Ro Khanna, in this effort to reform healthcare delivery at the state level will allow conservatives to finally have something to offer on the sentinel domestic policy issue of our time.

Conservatives who support state-based health-system reform with better care and simpler financing are demonstrating their commitment to constitutional governance, biblical principles, and fiscal responsibility. Better private healthcare delivery with unified and simpler public health financing are the constituents of health-system reform that allows for better, simpler, cheaper care shared equally by all American patients. It is both progressive in the Teddy Roosevelt sense and conservative in the original American sense. And it is how this nation can heal itself from the divisive and increasingly violent ugliness into which national discourse has deteriorated. We will not stay mad at each other if we are actively seeking to care for one another. The New Testament has it right, for when we heal "the lame, the maimed, the blind, the mute, and many others," when we visit the sick and injured, even the least of them, we will be invited into a new kingdom, a regime on the right hand of God, or, for some, on the right side of history.

9

HARRIS WOFFORD, FORCE, AND HARSHNESS

Thirty years ago, when I was first becoming acquainted with the strength of the published health-policy literature that supports better, simpler, and therefore cheaper health-system reform, I was persuaded by political events in Pennsylvania that the nation was preparing to elect leadership that would bring about the needed health-system changes. In 1991, then Democratic governor of Pennsylvania, Robert Casey, was in search of someone who could immediately assume the United States Senate seat from the Keystone State, a seat vacated when Senator John Heinz was killed in an aviation accident over a schoolyard in the Philadelphia suburbs. And then, while serving as United States Senator, the appointee would need to run a campaign to keep the seat opposing Dick Thornburgh, the still-popular, former, two-term Republican governor who had preceded Casey.

After some searching and even offering the opportunity to former Chrysler executive Lee Iacocca, Governor Casey announced the appointment of Harris Wofford, who, despite serving at the time as Pennsylvania Labor and Industry Secretary, was an unknown and a first-time candidate. Wofford had served on the staff of John F. Kennedy's presidential campaign and enjoyed some success in bringing African-American voters to support the Democratic ticket for the first time. He went on to participate in the founding of the Peace Corps in the Kennedy administration.

Because he was a novice running against a veteran politician who had the backing of President George H. W. Bush, who was then basking in high popularity after the successful prosecution of the first war against Iraq, Wofford was given no chance of winning the special election. The first poll taken in the very short campaign had Thornburgh, then serving as the attorney general of the United States, up by forty-seven points.

Wofford gamely took on the domestic policies of the first Bush administration and, noting that the economy was in recession with middle-class anxiety rising, he stumbled on a line that repeatedly gave him the applause he craved: "The Constitution says that if you are charged with a crime, you have a right to a lawyer. But it's even more fundamental that if you're sick, you should have the right to a doctor." Wofford rode that line and the Pennsylvania public's craving for health care security to a 55 to 45 percent win, a totally unexpected political victory that sent shock waves through the nation. For the first time, it appeared the American public had an appetite for health-system reform.

Wofford later said, "Until I had that victory, people weren't seeing [health care] as the big issue. And [Bill] Clinton called me the day after I was elected. . . . [H]e hadn't settled on health care as a big campaign issue." Clinton apparently considered placing Wofford on the Democratic ticket with him in the summer of 1992, and he ended up making health-system reform a central part of his winning campaign. After taking office, Clinton famously turned health-system reform over to his spouse and a White House team charged with organizing the program, which became all federal government and more about coverage than care.

The defeat of Hillary Care spelled the end of Wofford's brief service in the United States Senate. He was defeated by Rick Santorum in 1994 as the Republicans took back both the House and Senate. Wofford later lamented the outcome of Clinton's misbegotten health-policy foray. He said: "The trouble was, after big promises, nothing came out. If we had had even the Children's Health Insurance Program [enacted in Clinton's second term] as a Step 1, which is the final compromise some of us were proposing, I think the victory for the Republicans, if they had it, would have been far less. If we just had something good to show for it. We had nothing. It was just a fiasco."

But in 1991, when Wofford came out of nowhere to win the special election, erasing a forty-point polling deficit, and change the national political conversation, it seemed to me that health-care reform could be a winning political strategy. The fact that Clinton botched that moment and ruined the chance for sustainable change then doesn't alter the observation that one well-placed United States Senate race can refocus the entire nation's political discourse.

The two presidents who succeeded President Clinton— George W. Bush and Barack Obama—both featured health reform prominently in their initial campaigns. Bush, contrary to typical Republican dogma, favored expanding Medicare to provide a medication benefit, and Obama spoke to increasing "coverage." They'd both learned from the "Hillary Care" debacle and left the sausage-making legislative details to Congress, where the medical-industrial complex easily owned the process and made sure that profiteering as business as usual in American health care thrived. In his first presidential campaign, even Trump nodded to the necessity of supporting public financing of health care with his against-the-Republican-grain promise to not "reform" Medicare by narrowing its benefits even while promising to repeal Obamacare. By the time he ran for reelection, Trump's empty promises on health care were simply not believable for the average voter.

Politicians from both major parties are vulnerable to health care insurgencies because both parties pander to the profiteering of the medical-industrial complex. Voters in the United States need to support candidates who offer the only constitutional and sustainable health-system reform solution—state-based, single-payer reform—whether or not those candidates are completely in alignment with all or some of the voters' other policy positions. Voting for state-based, single-payer health-system reform will likely require changing party support or candidate choices "even from election to election." We American voters need to jettison our partisan voting patterns and consistently throw out members of Congress and legislatures, presidents and governors, who do not put patients before profits. I stand by my election dogma: every voter in the United States should begin each election cycle with a bias against incumbents because they have already proven themselves unable to do the right thing for American patients.

Progressives who have long sought a national single-payer Medicare for all need to use the middle of the road on this issue and agree to invite conservative voters to the health-reform table by offering state-based health reform as the viable political alternative, as Representative Ro Khanna has done. The Wofford effect proves that there is a latent desire across the American electorate to really make progress and solve our nation's health-system woes. Nothing will get the attention of Congress more than refusing to elect an incumbent of either major party over his or her failure to act sustainably and in patients' interest on health care.

The Child Health Insurance Program, or CHIP, is a prime example of how state-based health policy can bring progressives and conservatives together. After the Clinton administration botched the Wofford moment and Hillary Care failed (for both political and unsound policy reasons), Senator Ted Kennedy (D-

MA) joined Senator Orrin Hatch (R-UT) to find a way to finance health care for children whose families were unable to afford it but were too well off to qualify for Medicaid. They proposed to fund the $20 billion federal expense for the new program by levying a tax on cigarettes, which generated pushback from the tobacco industry, leading to initial legislative failure. Senator Trent Lott (R-MS), who was probably more concerned about the tobacco tax than the need to care for children, opposed the proposal on the basis that it was another "big" government intervention in people's lives.

Senator Lott's concern for the tobacco lobby at the expense of the children of the American republic reminds me of another City Creek Canyon moment. After the flood in 1983, City Creek's sidewalls were washed out and needed rebuilding. Where the creek at its highest flood stage had washed out or undermined the road, creek bed and sidewall repair took the form of stone walls loosely held together with wire fencing.

About ten years after the flood, I was living in Colorado but visiting Salt Lake City with my family. We took the opportunity to picnic in the canyon one evening. About half a mile from the entry gate, we found a roadside picnic table and settled in for a delightful evening.

My four kids—Margaret, the youngest, was not born until a few years later—began exploring the creek. Suddenly, the summer serenity was interrupted by piercing screams from Caitlin, my fourth child, who was about five years old at the time. I ran immediately to her creek-side location about fifty yards from the picnic table where my wife and I had been sitting. A rattlesnake had emerged from the loose rock wall between the creek and road, and it was coiled and rattling with its head a foot away from Caitlin's face. I jumped from road level down the three-foot height of the loose-rock creek wall to where Caitlin stood, and in one motion picked her up and pulled her away from the snake. As we retreated, the snake did likewise, and the situation was immediately defused. We returned to our picnic table fifty yards away, Caitlin calmed down, and the evening once again became peaceful.

Pardon the simplistic metaphor, but there are rattlesnakes threatening our domestic tranquility here in the United States, and they often linger in the very institutions we have built to secure our blessings. These vipers will threaten our children merely because the interests of kids can sometimes interfere with a profitable business model, as was the case when a tax on cigarettes was proposed in a bipartisan fashion to fund health services for children who up until then did not have routine medical care. Our elected officials, as was the case at this legislative moment with Senator Lott, as often as not take up the cause of the rattlesnake, in effect becoming the senator from Big Tobacco, or Big Pharma, or whatever big corporate interest has currently purchased the attention of any particular member of Congress.

Unusually, in this case, Mr. Lott failed to carry the day because his objection was wrong on its face. CHIP, like Medicaid, was proposed as a shared state/federal program, not a massive new federal, big-government initiative or entitlement. In effect, CHIP is an invitation from the federal government for states to use the public, revenue-generating power of national government to fashion and implement policy to promote the general welfare of children within their own borders. Both progressives and original American conservatives can see value in that constitutionally blessed kind of governance. CHIP has been far more effective than either the Bush Medicare expansion or Obamacare both because it was bipartisan and because it was the proper constitutional mix of state and federal action.

The combination of federal financing and state implementation in the case of CHIP has worked to the advantage of children in the United States. Because of Medicare and CHIP, virtually all Americans older than sixty-five years of age and younger than eighteen have some form of healthcare financing.

A study of the effects of CHIP on the health of children published in 2018 states, in part:

> "[Prior to CHIP,] a substantial share of children remained uninsured: those whose families earned above incomes needed to qualify for Medicaid but lacked employer-sponsored coverage and those for whom private insurance remained unaffordable. . . . CHIP, which began in 1997, filled in the gap for families at these income levels. . . . Research using quasi-experimental methods has found that children who become eligible for public insurance through expansions in Medicaid or CHIP are more likely to see a doctor at least once a year, are more likely to be in better health as teenagers and as adults if they were eligible for public insurance while young, and have lower mortality as teens and adults."[1]

Obviously, my optimism about sustainable health-system reform thirty years ago has gone unfulfilled. The singular failure of the United States within the developed world to enact a health policy that actually cares for its people has occurred because the will of the people of the United States, who consistently articulate support for public financing for everyone's needed health care, is always subverted by the loyalty of elected politicians of both parties to the corporate special interests—the snakes I refer to as the medical-industrial complex. Sustainable, universal health policies are found in the several dozen other first-world economies. For decades, single-payer health-system reform has been studied repeatedly in the United States and is always shown to be more efficient and to offer potentially higher-quality care than business as usual in American for-profit healthcare delivery. The failure to enact sustainable health-system reform in the United States is not a policy failure; it is a political failure. Our elected representatives have repeatedly chosen to foster the interests of the rattlesnakes instead of the general welfare of Americans.

Old Testament prophets spoke out about exactly this kind of societal problem in Ezekiel 34:2–4:

> "Ah, you shepherds of Israel who have been
>   feeding yourselves! Should not shepherds feed
>   the sheep? You eat the fat, you clothe your-
>   selves with the wool, you slaughter the fatlings;
>   but you do not feed the sheep. You have not
>   strengthened the weak, you have not healed
>   the sick, you have not bound up the injured,
>   you have not brought back the strayed, you
>   have not sought the lost, but with force and
>   harshness you have ruled them."

I have spent three decades trying to advance the cause of state-based health-system reform leading to better quality privately delivered health care with unified, simpler public-sector financing. I have given hundreds of speeches all across the country; lobbied the legislatures in Nevada, Utah, and Colorado; met repeatedly with members of Congress from both parties, both at home and in Washington, DC; appeared on dozens of media broadcasts, both radio and TV; written and published dozens of op-ed pieces; participated in public debates; joined community efforts to examine health policy; run for office four times (usually as a Republican nominee); posted thousands of messages and links on social media outlets like Facebook and Twitter; formed a political-issue committee; started a nonprofit organization; traveled thousands of miles; met thousands of people; marched; protested; studied; taken dozens of business leaders to lunch; and written two books (including this one). I know there are literally thousands of people across the country who, like me, are making personal sacrifices to urge the country to adopt a better, sustainable health policy. Nonetheless, it's hard to avoid feeling like a lone voice in the wilderness, crying for justice and mercy like an Old Testament prophet seeking to bring the people of Israel back to God.

In fact, because of my many years' experience preaching about the need for health-system reform, I believe I am coming to better understand the prophet Jeremiah, who lived and prophesied for forty years in Jerusalem before the destruction of that city by the Babylonian army approximately six hundred years before the common era. As is true today, the Middle East in Jeremiah's time was a constantly boiling cauldron of regional interests fighting for control.

Jeremiah, who is thought to have been born into an elite, priestly family in Jerusalem, emerged as a spokesman for God during the reign of King Josiah more than six hundred years before Jesus of Nazareth was born. This was the time when the Assyrian kingdom, which had conquered and destroyed the Northern Kingdom of Israel, was imploding and leaving a power vacuum in the Middle East. King Josiah, one of the few righteous kings in the history of Jerusalem, tried both to reform his people and assert influence in what had been the Northern Kingdom of Israel, then no longer under foreign rule. He reoccupied Megiddo, a strategic site along the main road between Egypt and Mesopotamia, where Babylon was on the rise.

Back in the days of King David, Megiddo was a main fortress for his military defense against Egypt and whatever kingdom was on the rise in Mesopotamia. But King Josiah simply didn't have the military wherewithal to intimidate either Egypt or Babylon; his country was weakened from within by a failure to live their best lives and care for each other.

Josiah died defending his country at Megiddo against an Egyptian invasion, and his brother Jehoiakim was placed on the Judean throne as a vassal of the Egyptian Pharaoh. The Egyptians, in turn, were defeated at Carchemish by the Babylonians, who then turned on Judea. Like his brother, Jehoiakim simply did not have a society strengthened by attention to integrity and mutual care. Jeremiah put it this way (NSRV):

> "You shall say to them, Thus says the Lord:
> When people fall, do they not get up again?
> If they go astray, do they not turn back?
> Why then has this people turned away
> in perpetual backsliding?
> They have held fast to deceit,
> they have refused to return.
> I have given heed and listened,
> but they do not speak honestly;
> no one repents of wickedness,
> saying, 'What have I done!'
> 'The harvest is past, the summer is ended,
> and we are not saved.'
> For the hurt of my poor people I am hurt,
> I mourn, and dismay has taken hold of me.
> Is there no balm in Gilead?
> Is there no physician there?
> Why then has the health of my poor people
> not been restored?"
> (Jeremiah 8: 4–6, 20–22)

Jeremiah went on hurting for his people for forty years, eventually witnessing the utter destruction of Jerusalem by the Babylonian army after a siege that caused a famine so severe that mothers ate their children's flesh. Jerusalem was burned to the ground, everything of value was plundered, and tens of thousands of its inhabitants were taken as slaves to work on the vast public projects in Babylon, which included two of the seven wonders of the ancient world: the massive wall around Babylon and the hanging gardens in the center of the city.

Unlike Jeremiah, I don't claim to speak for God. But with him, I lament that my fellow citizens hold fast to deceit and do not speak honestly. I wonder why my nation cannot seem to get health-system reform done well but rather turns away from what is known to best serve our patients and instead perpetually backslides into avaricious schemes. No wonder we have begun to hate each other, divide ourselves into political tribes, and justify violence as a means to a political end.

As does Jeremiah, I ask, "Why then has the health of my poor people not been restored? Is there no balm in Gilead? Is there no physician there?" Just as Jeremiah surely knew, we know there is a balm in Gilead. We know how to make it possible for physicians to care for patients. But we perpetually backslide into avarice. For the hurt of my people, I am hurt.

Business as usual in American health care causes pain and suffering of biblical proportions. Reasonable estimates indicate that 250,000 or more Americans die each year due to preventable injuries sustained through poor hospital practices. Another 50,000 die because, despite being taxed more for health care than the citizens of any other country, tens of millions of Americans have no financing for needed health care.

Imagine, in the richest country in the history of the world, people who suffer appendicitis can and do die because they do not have enough money to pay for a simple abdominal surgery. Diabetic patients pass away because they cannot afford insulin. Cancer patients can't afford the parking fees charged to them at some of the high-profile cancer centers in our country, much less the expensive treatments they need to assuage pain or, hopefully, cure the cancer. The Go Fund Me website is dominated by patients asking for funds for needed treatment. Children hold bake sales to raise funds to offset their loved ones' healthcare costs.

Meanwhile, in the struggle to pay for needed health care, millions of Americans—after being taxed more heavily for health care than is the case in any other country—are bankrupted by the cost of needed care for illness or injury. healthcare costs are bankrupting American government at all levels, federal, state, and local. As the portion of the gross domestic product devoted to health care continues to rise, we as a people are less able to support infrastructure, educate children, put nutritious food on the table, pay a living wage, house ourselves, and give people an honest chance in life. High healthcare costs lock people into less-productive jobs. healthcare costs can now dominate a household budget so severely that home ownership is impossible. Good jobs go fleeing across our borders because employers are seeking good health care for employees at a reasonable cost.

The business model of healthcare delivery in the United States prevents the pursuit of life, liberty, and happiness by many average Americans. Meanwhile, the medical-industrial complex makes bank and then makes it again and again. And they are supported in this profiteering by politicians from both major political parties who deceive us, the voters, time and again. Why does the electorate of the United States hold fast to this deceit and not demand that our political leaders speak with integrity? Why then has the health of my poor people not been restored? Is there no balm in Gilead? Is there no physician there? For the hurt of my poor people, I am hurt.

10

DOWNSTREAM DANGER

The flood of City Creek Canyon fails as a proper allegory for the biblical deluge of misery that is the relentless result of business as usual in American health care, where "providers" would rather make a sale than care for a patient. No one died in the City Creek Canyon flood of 1983. Damage was done, but not so much that it changed anything that really mattered in Utah's economy. I turn to Pennsylvania, the state that spawned the Wofford moment, for a flood of proper biblical proportion to serve as an analogy for the massive waste of human life and treasure that is our modern American healthcare system.

On May 31, 1889, a sixty-foot wall of water smashed into Johnstown, Pennsylvania, an industrial town with thirty thousand residents on the west side of the Allegheny Mountains. More than two thousand people died that afternoon, a flood death toll greater than all other such events in American history with the exception of two hurricanes. Cost estimates for the damage inflicted by the flood place the value at about $20 billion in 2020 dollars. David McCullough, an award-winning American historian, wrote a definitive account of the Johnstown flood, from which the following excerpts are extracted:

> "Most of the people in Johnstown never saw the water coming; they only heard it; and those who lived to tell about it would for years after try to describe the sound of the thing as it rushed on them. . . . Everyone heard shouting and screaming, the earsplitting crash of buildings going down, glass shattering, and the sides of houses ripping apart. . . . Those who actually saw the wall of water would talk and write of how it "snapped off trees like pipestems" or "crushed houses like eggshells" or picked up locomotives (and all sorts of other immense objects) "like so much chaff.". . . Because of the speed it had been building as it plunged through Woodvale, the water struck Johnstown harder than anything it had encountered in its fourteen-mile course from the dam. . . . The drowning and devastation of the city took just about ten minutes. For most people they were the most desperate minutes of their lives, snatching at children and struggling through the water, trying to reach the high ground, running upstairs as houses began to quake and split apart, clinging to rafters, window ledges, anything, while the whole world around them seemed to spin faster and faster. But there were hundreds, on the hillsides, on the rooftops of houses out of the direct path, or in the windows of tall buildings downtown, who just stood stone-still and watched in dumb horror."[1]

McCullough goes on to describe the pileup of debris that became lodged against a stone railroad bridge downstream from Johnstown, sealing off the flow of water for several hours and then catching fire. Hundreds of people were trapped in the debris, most of whom were able to escape either on their own or with the help of other survivors. The fire burned all night, with an estimated eighty people who had somehow survived the rampaging water tragically perishing in the conflagration. The smell of burning flesh permeated the Johnstown area all night long. Survivors were mostly huddled, wet and chilled, without shelter wherever they had managed to climb to get out of the deluge. Separated by the flood from family and friends, they did not know what they would find when they were able to search the next day.

The cause of the flood was the failure of an earthen dam. Originally proposed in 1838 and completed fifteen years later as part of a canal system meant to bring the state of Pennsylvania into transport competition with New York and the Erie Canal, the coming of the railroads soon after the completion of the canal rendered the dam and reservoir irrelevant. Eventually, the reservoir was repurposed as a recreational lake by what became known as the South Fork Fishing and Hunting Club, an exclusive, private enterprise catering to the very wealthy in Pittsburgh, eighty miles away.

The dam was nine hundred feet across and seventy-two feet high above the South Fork Creek on the downstream side. Lake Conemaugh, the name given the reservoir behind the dam, was usually about six or seven feet below the top of the dam and stretched two miles upstream. McCullough estimated that "the lake covered about 450 acres and was close to seventy feet deep in places," with the total water content weighing about twenty million tons.

Originally, there were five cast-iron pipes, each two feet across, designed to release water from the lake as needed for canal filling or relieving excess lake water. The dam had failed in 1862 but with minor damage since the lake had been only half filled at the time. However, at the time of this first dam failure or soon thereafter, the tower that controlled the water release through the pipes caught fire and burned to the ground.

During the 1870s, the owner pursued the cheapest plan to repair the dam: simply fill in the breach, restoring the dam to its original height. The repair process started with closing off the stone culvert meant to release water as needed and dumping whatever was at hand into the breach, including rocks, mud, brush, tree boughs, hay, and horse manure. The discharge pipes were not replaced. In what should have been seen as a harbinger of bad things to come, heavy rains twice washed out the repair work. As a consequence, during the 1880s, there were frequent rumors about the dam's imminent demise, to the point that people started paying little attention to them.

The general disregard for the dam's poor condition remained in force despite the fact that a competent engineering report filed about the dam in 1880 read in part:

"There appear to me two serious elements of danger in this dam. First, the want of a discharge pipe to reduce or take the water out of the dam for needed repairs. Second, the unsubstantial method of repair, leaving a large leak, which appears to be cutting the new embankment. As the water cannot be lowered, the difficulty arises of reaching the source of the present destructive leaks. At present there is forty feet of water in the dam, when the full head of 60 feet is reached, it appears to me to be only a question of time until the former cutting is repeated. Should this break be made during a season of flood, it is evident that considerable damage would ensue along the line of the Conemaugh. It is impossible to estimate how disastrous this flood would be, as its force would depend on the size of the breach in the dam with proportional rapidity of discharge. The stability of the dam can only be assured by a thorough overhauling of the present lining on the upper slopes, and the construction of an ample discharge pipe to reduce or remove the water to make necessary repairs."[2]

The wealthy Pittsburgh owners of the South Fork Fishing and Hunting Club who ignored this report and thought only about their convenience and pleasure while spending as little as possible to retain water for their private lake, bear significant responsibility for the heavy loss of life and treasure on May 31, 1889, though no court ever held them liable.

The flood immediately captured the attention of the nation. Newspaper reports were updated continuously, with new editions of the papers coming out hourly. Within twenty-four hours of the flood, at a mass meeting about the urgency of sending aid to Johnstown held in Pittsburgh, more than $48,000 in cash was collected for the flood victims. The first trainloads of supplies arrived in Johnstown later that same day. Ultimately, the people of Pittsburgh gave $560,000. McCullough records that the generosity came from across the nation:

> "New York City gave $516,000, Philadelphia, $600,000; Boston, $150,000. Nickels and dimes came in from school children and convicts. Churches sent $25, $50, $100. In Salt Lake City thousands of people turned out for a concert given in the huge Mormon Tabernacle, the proceeds of which were sent to Johnstown. . . . Tiffany & Company sent $500. R. H. Macy & Company sent $1,000. Joseph Pulitzer sent $2,000; Jay Gould, $1,000; John Jacob Astor, $2,500. The New York Stock Exchange gave $20,000. . . . Money poured in from every state and from fourteen countries overseas. . . . In all, the contributions from within the United States would come to $3,601,517.80. The sum from abroad was $141,300.98 . . . and this does not include the goods of every kind that rolled in by the trainload."[3]

Volunteers came in great numbers, but as McCullough notes:

> "The most resilient worker of them all, and certainly the one who stirred up the most talk, was a stiff-spined little spinster in a plain black dress and muddy boots who had brought the

newly organized American Red Cross in from Washington. Miss Clara Barton and her delegation of fifty doctors and nurses had arrived on the B & O early Wednesday morning [June 5, 1889]. . . . [O]nce there [in Johnstown] she knew that her Red Cross had arrived at its first major disaster. The organization, she had long argued, was meant for just such emergencies, and now she intended to prove it. . . . Hospital tents were to be opened immediately, construction was to start on temporary "hotels" for the homeless, and a house-to-house survey was to be conducted to see just how many people needed attention. . . . Within a very short time several large tents were serving as the cleanest, best-organized hospitals in town; six Red Cross hotels, two stories tall, with hot and cold running water, kitchens, and laundries, had been built with some of the fresh lumber on hand. . . . When the survey was completed it was found that a large number of people with serious injuries had been too weak or broken in spirit to do anything to help themselves. . . . Clara and her people did their best to tend everyone they could. Clara herself worked almost round the clock, directing hundreds of volunteers, distributing nearly half a million dollars' worth of blankets, clothing, food, and cash. . . . She stoutly proclaimed that the Red Cross was there to stay as long as there was work to do. . . . Clara stayed for five months, never once leaving the scene even for a day. . . . The Red Cross had clearly arrived."[4]

Today's American healthcare system deluges Americans with hurt and harm inflicted by a business model that amasses massive profits while wreaking havoc on human lives. The medical-industrial complex robs the American people through financial waste and ruin equal to the financial damages of the Johnstown flood every ten days. Every three days of business as usual, American health care kills the same number of Americans as lost their lives in the Johnstown flood.

Beyond the actual cost and loss of life is the devastation dealt by the business model of American health care to American patients and their families. Americans work hard but are commonly unable to afford the care they or their family members need, even if they are "covered" by health insurance. For most Americans today, the most desperate times of their lives will be when serious illness or injury happen and they discover they have no financing for the needed care. Like the Johnstown flood victims, they will huddle for financial shelter wherever they can but without knowing whether they or their loved ones can possibly survive without the needed medical intervention.

What American politicians have allowed to happen to American patients in the name of market-based medicine amounts to a plague of biblical proportions. Jeremiah's words can have no better application in modern times than as a descriptor of the agony of Americans who faithfully pay taxes but receive, at best, mediocre and often *no* healthcare services: "For the hurt of my poor people I am hurt, I mourn, and dismay has taken hold of me. Is there no balm in Gilead? Is there no physician there? Why then has the health of my poor people not been restored?" (Jeremiah 8:20–22).

The health of the American people has not been restored, because wealthy men and women, the owners and proprietors of the medical-industrial complex, are enriching themselves with our healthcare taxes, premiums, copayments, deductibles, coinsurance, and point-of-service payments. They are writing the rules by which they secure optimal profit at the least effort and expense to themselves.

Like the wealthy owners of the South Fork Fishing and Hunting Club, they are ignoring the downstream dangers of their business model. Unlike the Johnstown flood, which only happened once, the deluge of harm and havoc from American health care kills a Johnstown flood equivalent twice each week, fifty-two weeks each year, and saps a Johnstown flood equivalent of wasted wealth from the American economy three times each month.

In 1889, the year of the Johnstown flood, the Pittsburgh skyline was a silhouette of steelmaking attesting to the source of wealth of the owners of the South Fork Fishing and Hunting Club who bear responsibility for the flood. Today, Pittsburgh's skyline is once again testament to the enormous wealth of the corporate interests combining to harm the inhabitants of western Pennsylvania, though now it is the medical-industrial complex that perpetrates the hurt and haunts the skyline.

We don't need the medical-industrial complex to organize the care required by American patients. We already tax ourselves enough to pay for high-quality, efficiently financed health care for every American who needs it. We, the American people, have the inherent goodness and good sense to organize the necessary enterprise for health care. Much like the national response to the Johnstown flood, we Americans rise to assist our loved ones, friends, neighbors, and fellow citizens, and even strangers, when they have illness and injury and need help. We have been generously taxing ourselves for decades to build hospitals, train doctors and nurses, shed the light of clinical science on new treatments, and organize the proper delivery of care.

The best care is the care that relies on the native altruism of our people. Like Clara Barton in the aftermath of the Johnstown flood, we Americans stay on the job as long as work needs to be done. We need to elect political leaders who will reflect this native goodness and remove the rent-seekers and profiteers who have been inserted into the care of our sick and injured.

Neither major political party is currently worthy of our trust when it comes to health care. Voters need to ignore their own historical party affiliations. From now on, we should vote only for those who will act in the interests of our patients. We must look carefully at each candidate, setting aside any party affiliation, and demand a Harris Wofford moment with each election cycle.

Western Pennsylvania is home to a second monument to a massive disaster in American history. Less than twenty road miles southeast from Johnstown, the Flight 93 National Memorial commemorates the determined efforts of forty patriotic Americans to thwart the plans of suicide terrorists to fly a Boeing 757—United Flight 93—into the United States Capitol Building on September 11, 2001. On that day, three other hijacked airplanes were flown into targeted buildings in New York City and Washington, DC, killing nearly three thousand people—just a few hundred more than died in the Johnstown flood.

It was the largest death toll due to enemy attack on American soil in the history of our country. All four of the planes were scheduled for nonstop, cross-country trips from east to west, meaning they would be full of fuel after takeoff, allowing for maximum explosive impact upon hitting buildings on the East Coast.

The first three planes each took off on time and within minutes hit their intended targets. At 8:46 a.m., Flight 11 hit the North Tower of the World Trade Center. At 9:03 a.m., Flight 175 hit the South Tower of the World Trade Center. And at 9:37 a.m., Flight 77 hit the Pentagon.

Flight 93 was delayed by congested air traffic for more than twenty-five minutes. By the time the hijackers took over the aircraft, the two World Trade Center collisions had occurred. When passengers on Flight 93 contacted their families to describe the hijacking of their plane, they were informed of the coordinated terrorist attacks underway and fully understood the implications for them. They probably did not know what the target was for their own flight, but they decided to prevent the enemy from completing its mission and threw themselves into the battle after the hijackers brought the plane around into an easterly flight path.

When it appeared to the hijackers that they would likely lose control of the plane, they chose to crash it into the ground rather than give the passengers a miracle victory of retaking and somehow landing the plane. At 10:03 a.m. on September 11, 2001, Flight 93 nosedived into an empty field in western Pennsylvania a mere twenty minutes flying time away from Washington, DC. Recovered evidence indicates that the target for the Flight 93 terrorists was the Capitol Building, where Congress was in session.

The passengers on Flight 93 are heroes and patriots because they are exemplars of American goodness and determination. Like the thousands of Americans who responded to the Johnstown flood with donations of dollars, goods, and services and who worked tirelessly for months thereafter to relieve distress, these forty Americans did for the rest of us what was needed and what only they could do. This is the native altruism of the American people. If we can manage to deploy it, we can fix everything wrong with our nation today, including our toxic healthcare system.

"For the hurt of my poor people I am hurt, I mourn, and dismay has taken hold of me. Is there no balm in Gilead? Is there no physician there? Why then has the health of my poor people not been restored?" (Jeremiah 8:20–22). Just as Jeremiah knew there really was a balm in Gilead and a physician to put it into practice, I know the balm we need in the United States today is within each of us.

Those who attacked the United States Capitol on January 6, 2021, in an effort to overturn a free and fairly conducted election in the name of the then-incumbent president disgraced the symbolic center of the republic the "Flight 93 Forty" died to save. Mr. Trump and the minions who want him to consider another run at the White House are not making anything great in America; they are tearing away the fabric of the American way of life. Partisanship is not patriotism. Trumpism has nothing to do with original American conservatism; rather, it is a conspiracy to eliminate the rule of law and replace it with a dictatorship.

The entire premise of today's Republican Party is nothing but the promotion of the personal interests of politicians. The Democratic Party, beholden as it is to monied special interests, has been too weak to rid the republic of the horrific influence of Trumpism. As President Eisenhower said, "If a political party does not have its foundation in the determination to advance a cause that is right and that is moral, then it is not a political party; it is merely a conspiracy to seize power.[5]" Both parties are guilty; members of both parties in Congress need to be replaced.

11

THE BELL TOLLS FOR EVERY AMERICAN

W e must strive to heal the nation by promoting the general welfare through a state-based, health-system reform characterized by improved quality private-sector healthcare delivery and simplified, unified public-health financing. Those members of Congress who stand in the way of enacting the super waiver legislation needed to free states to make better use of the vast public funding already flowing into American health care are choosing avarice instead of altruism. We need a Harris Wofford moment to rid our Congress of these rattlesnake servants. The progressive electorate, some of whom are already listed among the sponsors of the needed legislation, will join conservatives in this task.

What we need is a way to tangibly and reliably care for ourselves. We need to put hands on each other and reach out to heal. "With malice toward none" and "charity for all,"[1] we need to visit even the least of our brothers and sisters. Dr. Edward Delos Churchill, a surgeon at Massachusetts General Hospital said, "Charity in the broad spiritual sense—the desire to relieve suffering . . . is the most precious possession of medicine.[2]" That is our way forward.

No matter which faction or tribe any one of us might adhere to, no matter how unfairly treated we each perceive ourselves individually to be, no matter how unloved or unloving we might be, we can offer the balm of Gilead to one another. We can choose to wrest the ownership of health care away from the medical-industrial complex and restore it to its original purpose —to act with charity in every American life.

We need no new appropriations; we have long since taxed ourselves heavily for health care. The public revenue streams already exist. Paraphrasing President Truman, we must simply decide that a "principal concern of the people of the United States is the creation of conditions of enduring" health.[3]

In fact, tens of thousands of us are already hard at work to restore the health of our people. In June 2019, I was invited to speak at the annual conference of Health Care for All Oregon (HCAO) held in Eugene, Oregon. HCAO is a consortium of thousands of individuals and hundreds of organizations and businesses who have the common goal of bringing about equitable, affordable, comprehensive, high-quality, publicly funded health care.[4]

Following is what I said to them. (I later gave much of this speech in front of the San Francisco home [located on Billionaires Row] of Nancy Pelosi, Speaker of the U.S. House of Representatives.)

Dr. John Symynges was one of London's most successful physicians in the late sixteenth century. He housed his family in upscale Cheapside, on Trinity Lane. He was wealthy, holding property in three counties, and was widely respected throughout town. He was a senior member of the Royal Academy of Medicine. It is said he owed all of this to his shrewd business sense. His mantra for his medical practice was simple: "Before you meddle with [a patient,] make your bargaine wisely now he is in paine." Quite simply, he urged fledgling doctors to settle the fee for treatment while the patient was unable to really negotiate.

Dr. Symynges and his self-serving style of practicing the business of medicine, despite his preeminence during his own lifetime, would be entirely forgotten to us now, and deservedly so, but for the accident of history that by marriage he became the stepfather of John Donne, one of England's greatest poets. John Donne received training in the law and later in life took holy orders and became the dean of St. Paul's, where he served for the last decade of his life. By this time in his life, Donne had already become more famous than his stepfather because of his poetry. However, the sermons and meditations he penned while a clergyman sealed his enduring fame. Once while too ill to arise from bed, he heard the church bell tolling and wrote his seventeenth Meditation:

"Perchance he for whom this bell tolls may be so ill, as that he knows not it tolls for him; and perchance I may think myself so much better than I am, as that they who are about me, and see my state, may have caused it to toll for me, and I know not that. . . . The bell doth toll for him that thinks it doth. . . . No man is an island, entire of itself; every man is a piece of the continent, a part of the main. If a clod be washed away by the sea, Europe is the less, as well as if a promontory were, as well as if a manor of thy friend's or of thine own were: any man's death diminishes me, because I am involved in mankind, and therefore never send to know for whom the bell tolls; it tolls for thee. . . Another man may be sick, too, and sick to death, and this affliction may lie in his bowels, as gold in a mine, and be of no use to him; but this bell, that tells me of his affliction, digs out and applies that gold to me, if by this consideration of another's danger I take mine own into contemplation."

Here we have an entirely different approach to the possibilities that contact with illness provides than that of the opportunistic practitioner. For Donne, illness in another, no matter how remote our contact, is to be shared, contemplated, and learned from. Wealth generated from the sick comes not as coin but as shared human experience for which the observer can be grateful. Applied to my professional life in clinical care, Donne's words signal me to accept my calling as a requirement to subsume my self-interest and seek to attach myself to a cause greater than my own because I am involved in mankind. Donne would have each of us contemplate our personal danger as we make ourselves aware of the afflictions of others.

These lessons of three hundred years ago need relearning now. Medicine, once again, has been reduced to a business opportunity. In a nation where tens of millions have no financing for basic healthcare services, leading to tens of thousands of preventable deaths annually, our body politic has become paralyzed by a market-oriented health policy. Bells are tolling, yet we pretend we are not diminished by the suffering of our fellow countrymen. We pretend that the afflictions of the uninsured are not ours to share, as if we individually are an island, entire of itself. This despite the fact that we pay twice as much per capita for health care than do the citizens of the rest of the developed world, mostly in the form of the highest per-person taxes for health care in the world. What we are missing is the contemplation of our own danger. Americans are least likely in the developed world to avoid death answerable to health care. We have allowed the business of medicine to so deviate our health system from its principal mission that preventable injury to hospitalized patients has become the third leading cause of death in our country.

More than twenty years ago, Tony Snow, who died from colon cancer while serving the Bush White House as press secretary, made this statement: "In the real world, people stampede when somebody slaps up a sign that reads 'free.' This is the theory behind bargain basements, but it also applies to hip replacements and appendectomies."

This is Dr. Symynges's approach to medicine reiterated in modern parlance, and it makes no more sense now than it did then. I have never met a patient willing to have his appendix removed because a hospital had bargain-basement appendectomies for sale. I doubt Mr. Snow actually behaved this way when he was a patient. As far as I know, Mr. Snow did not attempt to start his course of chemotherapy before he had cancer because he found the drugs on sale. After colon cancer, would he still maintain that Dr. Symynges's approach to making the bargain with the patient while he is yet in pain is the correct one? Is medicine a commodity, efficiently traded and distributed by markets? Are patients shoppers or customers, or are they the people for whom the bell tolls?

The Wall Street Journal, an authority on markets and customers, may help us with an answer. A few years ago, an opinion piece in the *Journal* included this thought:

> "Research at Dartmouth Medical School suggests that if everyone in America went to the Mayo Clinic, our annual healthcare bill would be 25% lower (more than $500 billion), and the average quality of care would improve. . . . Of course, not everyone can get treatment at Mayo. . . . But why are these examples of efficient, high quality care not being replicated all across the country? The answer is that high quality, low-cost care is not financially rewarding. Indeed, the opposite is true. Hospitals and doctors can make more money providing inefficient, mediocre care."[5]

If the statement that hospitals and doctors are paid to deliver inefficient, mediocre care confuses you, let me illustrate with data from a hospital in central Utah. In the mid-1990s, a family physician practicing at Sanpete Community Hospital observed that patients presenting for treatment of pneumonia were not receiving optimal care and therefore becoming sicker and dying more often than should have been the case. He organized a protocol for optimal treatment of community-acquired pneumonia, persuaded every one of his physician colleagues at the hospital to follow it, and induced the hospital to adopt it. Almost overnight, the care of pneumonia improved; 25 percent fewer patients became sick enough to require hospitalization. For those patients admitted to the hospital, the length of stay dropped by one-third. The length of time before the instigation of proper antibiotic treatment dropped by one-fourth. And the cost per case fell by one-half. This is the optimal outcome in a market: the quality of service goes up, and the cost drops by half.

In a functioning free market, the provider of such service would be handsomely rewarded. Unfortunately for Sanpete Community Hospital, there was no reward. In fact, the amount paid for pneumonia care fell even more than per case cost; the hospital took a financial hit for providing better treatment.

Hospitals and doctors get the best payments when they let their patients get as sick as possible. The business model of the medical-industrial complex, because of the for-profit motive, is more about making sales than caring for patients. This is what the *Wall Street Journal* meant when it said there are perverse incentives in the American healthcare system. The fact that American health care pays doctors to harm patients through mediocre care is evidence that market principles are not at work in health care. A market does not have perverse incentives. And a market commodity does not have a lower price for higher quality. Health care is not a commodity. Dr. Symynges was wrong; the best bargains are not driven by the patient's pain.

If you want further evidence that health care is not a market commodity, consider this: around $3 trillion of our nation's more than $4 trillion annual health economy comes from our taxes. What other market is two-thirds tax funded? Why do we taxpayers agree to fund health care with so much tax money? Because, in our hearts and minds, we know that John Donne is right—any man's death diminishes me. It matters to all of us whether the uninsured tuberculosis patient receives appropriate care; his illness places society at risk. In health care, we do not believe in *caveat emptor* because the buyer is a patient, neither prepared nor able to shop. We place ethical obligations on physicians to serve their patients' needs ahead of personal interests. John Donne was right: when it comes to health care, Americans have always known that no man is an island.

To be fair, it is not generally today's health professional who is manipulating the moment of need created by injury and illness to extract profit. Rather, doctors are commonly victimized along with their patients by the business model of American health insurance, illustrated by the following passage from the advertising literature of a California health insurer: "We believe that the cost of covering someone whose health can be predicted to require costly care should not be subsidized by someone with minimal health care needs. . . . All enrollments are subject to medical underwriting. We may change or terminate coverage . . . with 30 days prior written notice."

In any given year, 80 percent of healthcare costs are accrued by only 20 percent of the population. But that bell tolls for each of us because none of us has any way of knowing when illness or injury will strike within our family and place us within the costly highest quintile. If we have not forced change on the health-insurance business model before that happens in our own household, we will be isolated on an island, entire of itself, making our healthcare bargain while we are in pain. Again, half of all personal bankruptcies in the United States are caused by illness and injury. And again, half of the households driven to bankruptcy by medical costs had health insurance at the time the health problem occurred.

These two examples—Sanpete Community Hospital and the California health insurer—illustrate the two principal problems created by the modern American health business model: quality waste and inefficiency. The *Wall Street Journal* pointed out that if all Americans received the higher-quality care delivered routinely at the Mayo Clinic, we could save $500 billion to $750 billion per year as a nation.

In health care, unlike a commodity in a free market, higher quality costs less. Because as a nation we follow Tony Snow and pretend that health care is a market, where competition will drive better bargains, we get poor-quality health care in three ways: we are given inappropriate or unnecessary care; we are injured by the care we receive; and as often as not, we do not receive proven clinical interventions at the proper time.

The experience at Sanpete Community Hospital demonstrates that if all of a region's health professionals and institutions cooperate to solve a community health problem, they can deliver higher-quality care at a lower price by eliminating unnecessary surgery and patient injury and consistently getting care right the first time. This is how we can save up to $750 billion per year with quality improvement. But remember the poor reimbursement for improved pneumonia care at Sanpete Community Hospital, which illustrates that our health-financing system based on the health-insurance business model must also change, or the efforts of doctors and nurses to improve care will go unrewarded and therefore not be sustained.

Health insurers have a two-part business model: exclude the potentially ill from coverage and creatively deny benefits. Both parts of the business model are expensive and distract from patient-centered care. Credible estimates place excess costs for the health-insurance business model at $500 billion per year. Taken together, quality waste and inefficiency cost the American taxpayer about $1 trillion per year and at least 250,000 premature, preventable deaths.

There is another almost universally ignored cost of wasting $1 trillion each year on quality waste and inefficiency, and that is opportunity cost. What else could we be doing with that $1 trillion of wasted healthcare spending? As stated, health care is principally funded through taxation and therefore competes for revenues with other tax-funded enterprises, such as education. Because we spend a greater portion of our gross domestic product on health care than do other developed nations, we spend a lesser proportion on education. McKinsey and Co. released a report stating that if we had improved our education system over the past generation, our annual gross domestic product could be as much as $2 trillion larger.[6]

Our fiscal health is not the only thing hurt by this opportunity cost. Education is important to health itself. Ensuring that all Americans receive a high school education could prevent an estimated 240,000 deaths per year, more than eliminating homicide, auto accidents, and diabetes combined.

That is one opportunity cost of United States healthcare business as usual. Another is the effect of excess health spending on American business itself. As a nation, our businesses spend less on new-product development than do those in other first-world nations, in part because of ridiculous healthcare costs. American auto manufacturers have for years spent $1,200 per car more on health care than has been true of their competitors in Japan and Germany. How has that affected the viability of the American auto-manufacturing industry? The opportunity costs of healthcare spending in the United States threaten our tax base and economy and therefore our way of life.

Ten years ago, when I first publicly spoke about the contrast between the Dr. Symynges and John Donne paradigms for health care, the nation was witnessing the Congressional fight ending with the passage of the Patient Protection and Affordable Care Act. I knew then, as hopefully many more Americans know now, that Obamacare would make everything that was already bad about American health care worse for three reasons.

First, during the Obamacare debate and up to the present time, Congress was and is principally debating how to cover the uninsured, as if that is the principal problem of our health system. Should we have a public plan option? Should we expand Medicare or Medicaid? Should there be a mandate to buy health insurance? The issue was not and is not coverage; it is cost control—or, more specifically, waste elimination. Per-capita health spending in the United States is twice as high as in any other nation, and rising faster, because we waste up to one-third of our health spending on inefficiency and poor quality. For example, overhead in American hospitals is five times higher than in other first-world nations, and postoperative wound infections occur as much as ten times more often than should be the case, at an average cost of $14,000 per case.

Wasteful health-system spending is the direct and inherent result of the business models of American health corporations. What I call *waste*, they call *profit*. These corporations spend $1 million per member of Congress per year on lobbying to defend their business models, which is why the bill that became Obamacare was written by and for the medical-industrial complex. Politicians from both major political parties, red and blue, are equally guilty of the corporate welfare that supports America's wasteful healthcare delivery. Waste elimination will be the hallmark of sustainable health-system reform, and it won't happen until politicians, both red and blue, are unelected when they pander to the medical-industrial complex.

Second, Obama frequently stated that reform should build on what works, by which he meant employment-based health benefits. He often reassured those with insurance that they could keep the health benefits to which they were clinging. This continues to be the premise of those resisting real and sustainable health-system reform. Trouble is, nothing works; the whole system is dysfunctional. In other words, the Obamacare premise is wrong: employee health benefits are riddled with faults, including poor quality, rising costs, inadequate coverage, and ridiculously massive overhead. What good is an employment-based health benefit if the family can't afford to pay the deductible, coinsurance, or copayment? Why is it optimal for a family to have health insurance that guarantees financing for hospitalization if hospital care is fraught with the risk for injury and premature death?

Third, not only is the wrong issue being discussed with the wrong premise, but I believe that Washington, DC, will become the wrong venue for this discussion. I am not opposed to Medicare for All. I hope Senator Sanders succeeds and leads us all to healthcare nirvana. But we should all be prepared for the contingency that the movement to enact Medicare for All will fall short. After all, the current president of the United States, Joe Biden, has openly stated that he will veto any Medicare for All bill that comes to his desk.

If it does, there are both political and functional reasons to pursue state-based, single-payer health-system reform. Foremost among these is that the federal legislation enabling state-based, single-payer reform can potentially benefit from support across a much broader spectrum of elected officials. Mike Lee, perhaps the most conservative member of the United States Senate, represents my state, Utah. He has publicly voiced his support for federal legislation making state-based health reform with better private healthcare delivery combined with unified, simplified public-health financing possible.

Real and sustainable health-system reform legislation will be bitterly opposed by the medical-industrial complex in Congress and in state legislatures. Ballot initiatives may be the only viable pathway to the passage of better, simpler, and therefore cheaper health reform, and, of course, that is only possible at the state level.

Finally, the function of health systems has been historically regional, meaning mostly regulated at the state level. My home state of Utah has higher-than-average healthcare quality and therefore lower-than-average healthcare costs. Shouldn't Utah be allowed to play to that strength? And why shouldn't Louisiana, the state with the poorest-quality and therefore highest-cost health care, have the opportunity to learn from states that are succeeding? Justice Louis Brandeis once said that the states are the laboratories of democracy.

One way Congress can act on health care is to set a minimum national standard for state performance and then provide a pathway for states to exceed that standard through negotiation out of federal rules and restrictions. This kind of legislation was introduced to Congress in 2021 by Representative Ro Khanna (D-CA) and cosponsored by, among others, three Congressmen from Oregon. It was called the State Based Universal Health Care Act. A serious proposal, Senate Bill 770 has surfaced in Oregon, establishing a commission tasked to study how to transform Oregon healthcare delivery into a universal, low-overhead system. The state of New York is one Senate vote shy of passing its own better-quality, lower-overhead reform package. Activists in the state of Washington have begun collecting signatures to qualify their own version of state-based better and simpler health-system reform for the ballot. And why shouldn't Oregon, Washington, and New York have the opportunity to experiment with their own proposals?

We are currently witnessing a national discussion about our health system. This is the seventh time in sixty years that our nation has contemplated whether there might be a better way to finance and deliver the care of the sick and injured. This time will be different only if you and I make it so. No social-change movement in our history has faced such a well-financed lobby protecting the status quo.

The medical-industrial complex has the means to make its message heard. Wendell Potter, former health-insurance executive turned single-payer advocate, has said that what is written in health-insurance board rooms in the morning is on the tongues of members of Congress from both parties that afternoon. As currently constituted, the medical-industrial complex owns Congress. If we want change, we must change Congress.

The midterm election in 2018 made a small change in Congress. Recent analysis has shown that Democrats won the total popular vote in the House elections that year by 7 percentage points. Contrary to a commonly held opinion, this modest victory for Democrats cannot be ascribed solely, or even mostly, to a surge of new progressive voters coming to the polls. Rather, the most important change driving the outcome of the midterm vote was vote switching among the ninety-nine million people who voted in both 2016 and 2018. Put simply, the 2018 election changed the leadership of the House because millions of people who voted for Trump in 2016 changed their vote to Democrat in 2018. This is what I call "purple-world" voting.

Many people are not inherently partisan. They can be persuaded to vote for candidates of either party. But it isn't party-line voting that will further the cause of better, simpler, and therefore cheaper health-system reform. Rather, what is needed is voters who are informed about healthcare policy and care about it enough to select candidates, regardless of party, who are committed to making change happen.

Focus groups conducted by the Kaiser Family Foundation prior to the 2020 election indicated that in that year, health care would be at the top of voter priorities. Most voters currently don't understand what is meant by better health care financed more simply and don't see how it will help them navigate the health-insurance system and pay for services. This means we can't afford to focus only on progressive candidates and their supporters. We must broaden our audience to include these millions of people in the moderate center who are nonpartisan. Let me suggest how this can be done.

First, broaden the geography of the single-payer movement. We need to educate voters in suburban and rural America about how we can reform health care such that privately delivered care is better and more simply, publicly financed. Rural America has an enormous influence on Congressional election outcomes, particularly in the Senate. There are about fifty million Americans living in rural settings, and they tend to be more conservative. Better, simpler, and therefore cheaper care is fiscally, morally, and, if state-based, constitutionally the most conservative approach to health-system reform.

Rural voters will be particularly aware of the failings of market-based healthcare delivery. They live where the so-called healthcare market never has approached a semblance of function. Rural hospitals all over the nation are failing, and the leaders of rural healthcare facilities have not joined their urban/suburban colleagues in overt opposition to real and sustainable health-system reform. Rates of disabilities and injury mortality are higher in rural areas. Rural America is ripe for a message about healthcare reform.

Second, when we speak to rural and suburban voters, we need to focus the health-reform message on the essential issues— waste elimination, or cost control. Two-thirds of Americans believe that our health system is in crisis, but, perversely, the majority of Americans believe the care they personally receive is high quality. This is whistling in the dark. We all want to believe our doctors and nurses can somehow do what is best for us despite the obvious dysfunction of American health care. It is our job as advocates for sustainable change to clearly articulate that healthcare delivery in the United States is poor in quality and inefficiently financed. Americans don't tolerate poor safety practices in air travel, as witnessed by the recent Boeing 737 Max grounding. But according to the National Institutes of Health and Johns Hopkins University, poor patient-safety practices in American hospitals are causing 250,000 premature deaths per year—the equivalent of more than a plane crash a day. We need to bring the American electorate to a heightened sense of urgency in health-system reform.

Third, don't allow the message about health-system reform to be viewed as yet another plank of the progressive left. As important as other issues may be, health-system reform is not about education, climate change, immigration, gun control, or reproductive rights. Health-system reform is the key domestic issue of our day. All Americans will be better off if we can improve the quality of care typically delivered while reducing administrative waste and thereby sustainably making universal care a reality. Think of what this means: universal mental health services, universally available high-quality reproductive health care, and better arrangements for primary care in all communities. Progress on many fronts in American life will be more possible once we are no longer paying the opportunity cost of our broken healthcare system.

Fourth, and finally, speaking to more conservative audiences requires changing our jargon. For instance, let's not fight about whether health care is a human right. Many people who are moderate or conservative won't agree because, as I heard former Surgeon General C. Everett Coop say, the right to health care is nowhere enshrined in our Constitution. My response to this is commonly to point out that there is no right to asphalt in the Constitution either, but I can drive from my house to the White House on publicly funded roads. No one ever says that interstate highways are a system of socialist roads.

Another example: Many conservative people believe malpractice reform should be an essential feature of health reform. Even though malpractice reform will not really change what's wrong with American health care, I try to find common ground with these audiences. I agree that defensive medicine is, by definition, clinically inappropriate care, one of the three principal types of poor-quality care common in United States health-care business as usual. And I tell them how single-payer health-system reform will eliminate quality waste, including clinically inappropriate care.

A final example: When conservatives criticize national single-payer health-system reform as yet another government over-reach, I tell them that state-based health-system reform characterized by high quality, privately delivered care with unified, simplified public-health financing can be accomplished through establishing a nongovernmental payer. My proposal for health reform in Utah features the conversion of the Public Employees Health Plan, a nonprofit private trust fund that efficiently pays for health services for state, municipal, county, and other public employees, into a cooperative serving all residents in the state without growing state government.

Health spending is on an unsustainable trajectory, and the opportunity costs of $1 trillion in health-system waste every year are threatening our tax base, our education system, our businesses, and our way of life. If Congress fails to eliminate health-system waste, we must be prepared to do so through state government. Let us embrace our current opportunity to redeem our healthcare system and reject health care as a business opportunity. Remember, no man is an island, entire of itself. Every man is a piece of the continent, a part of the main. Never send to know for whom the bell tolls; it tolls for thee.

If I have persuaded you with the words I spoke to HCAO in 2019 and with the arguments I have made throughout this book that the time is ripe for each of us to rise up and realize the promise of national goodness and altruism and find a way to bind up our national wounds through sustainable health-system reform, then allow me to point you to your next step. It will not do for you to sit still and do nothing when the nation requires a massive political lift to overcome the vast resources of the medical-industrial complex. HCAO is only one of the dozens of state-based and local organizations diligently working toward the day when every American can receive the gift of health care when it is needed, without point-of-service cost.

One Payer States, a nationwide nonprofit coalition of state-based health-system-reform advocacy groups, lists twenty-one states with active movements working toward single-payer health-system reform. I urge you to connect to this massive and growing movement by visiting the website of One Payer States (onepayer-states.org) and find out what, if any, organization is already hard at work where you live, and join them. If you do not find a local contact on the One Payer States website, contact OPS directly and offer to join them. If what you need is information, OPS will provide it. If you have time to offer, OPS will use it. If you have money to donate, then join me in supporting the American Health Security Project, which is on the web at americanhealth-securityproject.org. The project has the exclusive purpose of picking and winning the political fights that will bring about needed and sustainable health-system reform. Here's what I said when I announced the formation of the project in early 2022:

Last summer during my trip to Washington, DC, to participate in the March for Medicare for All, I took the time to meet with two of the Congressmen who represent my state of Utah in the U.S. House of Representatives. Both of these men are Republicans, of course, since Utah is probably the most Republican state in the Union. These two conversations were different in some ways. Both men had taken some time to read portions of my book *The*

Purple World: Healing the Harm in American Health Care. One of the two was quite critical of the book, doubting most of the assertions that I made therein that U.S. patients suffer under a healthcare system that provides mediocre quality at a ridiculously high price. The other Congressman was more friendly to the idea that American health care needed attention. But what was the same was that both men aligned themselves with the **politics** of health-system reform and not its necessity or the facts of health-system failure. Both knew inherently that what I had to say was contrary to the interests of the medical-industrial complex, that group of for-profit corporate interests that owns and operates American healthcare delivery. Neither of these two Congressmen was interested in taking on the corporate healthcare complex because that is the largest source of campaign funds and lobbying might.

Given that I knew I was talking with Republicans, I did not approach those meetings expecting to persuade either Congressman to endorse single-payer health-system reform, America's only option for improving our care. Rather, I asked them to consider backing HR 3775, the State Based Universal Health Care Act, which is legislation intended to allow states to make comprehensive, sustainable health-system reforms. This bill has the backing of some progressive members of the U.S. House of Representatives. I asked each of these two men to consider becoming the first Republican sponsors of the bill and move the legislation toward a hearing. But here again, **politics** became the guiding sentiment for each of these Congressmen. They did not trust progressive members of Congress to offer legislation that was worthy of their attention, even if, in principle, each agreed that states should be where health-system reform should happen.

In my thirty years of health-system-reform advocacy, I have met with dozens of state and federal legislators and their staff members, offered testimony before many legislative committees in Nevada, Colorado, and Utah, and spoken to both democrat and republican platform committees, delegates, and interest groups. The results of these many encounters have been no different than this recent experience in Washington DC. **Politics**, meaning the alignment with party and special interests, is more important to elected officials than any human experience or set of facts. Those of us who are trying to change how Americans do healthcare business must recognize that health-system reform is about **POLITICS**. No amount of education or marching to draw attention to the plight of American patients will change the grip of the medical-industrial complex on business as usual in American health care. Health-system reform is first and foremost a very heavy political lift, meaning it is a power grab, meaning someone's ox must be gored. Members of Congress must learn that we mean business and that we are coming after their seats if they don't help make the changes necessary. We must pick political fights and win them.

To that end, I announce the formation of a new super PAC, or political action committee, called the American Health Security Project. I am joined on the steering committee of this new PAC by Lisa Theobald, Laura Fielding, and Georgia Davenport. Together we are building a political platform for a grassroots effort to hammer home the message first articulated in Congress by the late Senator John McCain. In 2017, after he received a diagnosis of terminal brain cancer, he returned to Congress to vote on the "skinny" repeal of Obamacare, which meant repeal but not replace. Republicans, then holding a slim majority in the United States Senate, had waited for his return before scheduling the vote because two Republican senators, Lisa Murkowski (R-AK) and Susan Collins (R-ME), had already declared their intent to vote against the "skinny" reform measure. But if McCain voted for it, a fifty-fifty tie could be realized, which would then be broken in favor of passage by Vice President Mike Pence. With the voting held open on the Senate floor, Senator McCain was personally lobbied by Mr. Pence and then took a call from President Trump in the cloakroom of the Senate. Despite those efforts, he returned to the floor of the Senate and voted against the bill, later stating:

> "Our healthcare insurance system is a mess. We all know it, those who support Obamacare and those who oppose it. Something has to be done. We Republicans have looked for a way to end it and replace it with something else without paying a terrible political price. We haven't found it yet. . . . The Obama administration and congressional Democrats shouldn't have forced through Congress without any opposition support a social and economic change as massive as Obamacare. And we shouldn't do the same with ours."

That will be the message of the American Health Security Project. American health care is a mess. Everyone knows it. Something beyond partisanship must be done about that mess. Politicians who support partisan measures like Obamacare and its skinny repeal are putting politics ahead of patient care. The American Health Security Project will hammer home the message that patients must come first, and members of Congress must join John McCain in voting for what is right, not what is politically partisan and expedient.

All Americans are health insecure. None of us knows whether the members of our families will have the funding and care needed to save lives and livelihoods. Democrats and Republicans alike have been successfully exploiting our health insecurities as the means to drive us apart from each other, divide us, and then win elections that allow each party in turn to govern us with force and harshness, denying us the care that we need. It is time to stop placing our time, efforts, and resources at the behest of either major political party when what we get in return is the indifference and posturing I have seen on Capitol Hill for thirty years.

I invite all Americans to change their political habits. If you routinely identify with either major party in the United States, instead of helping them, from now on, bring the dollars and the doing you usually donate to candidates and political causes to the American Health Security Project. We will swamp social media with the political speech that explains how horrible health insecurity is for all of us and articulates what we can do to make better, simpler, and therefore cheaper care available to all Americans, with no payments at the point of service. We Americans are taxing ourselves more for health care than do the citizens of any other nation, but Republican and Democratic politicians alike are giving these public resources away to the medical-industrial complex at the expense of our patients and our families. The American Health Security Project will fund state-level ballot initiatives across the nation that will revolutionize health care in our country. Together we can identify the particular politicians, red or blue, who stand in the way of real and sustainable health-system reform and, with the means of a grassroots super PAC, oust them. Unseating even one member of Congress because of his or her failure to protect patients will dramatically change the deportment of all the rest.

You can find the American Health Security Project online at https://americanhealthsecurityproject.org/. Take time today to go to that website and make a pledge of whatever time and fiscal resources you can spare to join us in pursuit of the massive political change needed to protect our patients. Once we have enough pledges to pay the expenses of the PAC for one year, we will ask you to convert the pledges to actual donations, and we will file the required documents and officially create the political-action committee. We will not accept donations from corporations. We will do our business as a grassroots organization, with open disclosure of how many donors and the total amounts received. We will not be partisan, but with the help of our donors, we will pick political fights and oppose those who harm our patients.

I'm tired of going to Congress, hat in hand, begging for

crumbs and receiving indifference or scorn. From now on, whatever funds I have to donate to American politics will go to the American Health Security Project, where I will join you in forging the hammer that will build consensus around caring for all Americans.

12

BIBLICAL WISDOM AND ORIGINAL AMERICAN CONSERVATISM

B efore referencing the biblical values that might help us meet this moment of division and hate in the not-so-United States, let me assure you, gentle reader, that I recognize that the Judeo-Christian tradition as articulated in the Bible is not the sole source of goodness, justice, and equity. I agree with President Eisenhower that "—under the American Constitution, under American tradition, and in American hearts, [Islam and by extension other belief or unbelief systems], is . . . welcome. . . . Indeed, America would fight with her whole strength for [the] right to have here [any] church. . . . This concept is indeed a part of America, and without that concept we would be something else than what we are."

I know the Bible because I was raised reading it and believing in the grace of God described therein. I am not as familiar with other books or documents that articulate the highest human aspirations or values, and I therefore cannot attempt to select passages from them to reflect meaning on our present national unhappiness. I seek to reference the Bible because that book is for many, beginning with me, a prime source of wisdom and inspiration.

Some people accept the Bible as the unerring word of God or scripture. Others view it as a collection of writings by human hands preserving some of the wisdom of a Semitic tribe that arose in the ancient Near East but also containing much that is unwise or unsupportable and nothing miraculous. I accept neither of those assessments as adequate for explication of my personal beliefs about the Bible because I find the Bible to be neither unerring nor un-miraculous.

In addition to my religious beliefs about the Bible, and more especially for purposes of this writing, I embrace the Bible as a foundational work of literature undergirding the aspirations of our nation's early leaders and therefore supporting what we Americans have come to live in our governance. The rule of law in the United States, for better or worse, can be understood to be a derivative of the Judeo-Christian tradition articulated in the Bible. Original American conservatism owes much to the King James translation of the Bible, the most-purchased book in the history of the world.

Here are some of the original American conservative values that can be found in the Bible and that I believe can lead us to a better place of understanding and save us from our selfish pride and consequent hatred of each other. For purposes of clarity and better understanding for the modern reader, I will quote from the translation known as the New Revised Standard Version of the Bible.

According to the Bible, the earliest admonitions to the nation of Israel by God through Moses were about essential societal functions. Moses was, according to the Old Testament, the founding prophetic voice of the people of the house of Israel, consisting of twelve tribes descended through the sons of Jacob, who was renamed Israel by God. As they left enslavement in Egypt 1,300 years before the common era, they were taught by God through Moses about how to conduct the business of their nation. In the book of Deuteronomy, the fifth and summary book of Moses, are the following passages:

> 1:17—You must not be partial in judging: hear out the small and the great alike; you shall not be intimidated by anyone, for the judgment is God's.

> 10:19—You shall also love the stranger, for you were strangers in the land of Egypt.

> 15:11—Since there will never cease to be some in need on the earth, I therefore command you, "Open your hand to the poor and needy neighbor in your land."

> 16:20—Justice, and only justice, you shall pursue, so that you may live and occupy the land that the Lord your God is giving you.

Clearly, the God of the people of Israel intended His people to govern with justice and with an eye to the welfare of all, whether poor, needy, ill, or from elsewhere. By extension, God means all nations to adopt a similar stance. The American Constitution, which was established in part to "promote the general welfare" and "establish justice," is clearly derivative from these biblical values.

The wisdom literature of the Bible, meant to inspire God's people to be their best selves both individually and as a nation, is also full of references to these principles needed to promote the general welfare and establish justice. Here are just a few examples:

Job 31:6—Let me be weighed in a just balance,
and let God know my integrity!

Psalm 7:8—Judge me, O Lord, according to my
righteousness and according to the integrity
that is in me.

Psalm 9:18—For the needy shall not always be
forgotten, nor the hope of the poor perish
forever.

Proverbs 3:29–31—Do not plan harm against
your neighbor who lives trustingly beside you.
Do not quarrel with anyone without cause,
when no harm has been done to you. Do not
envy the violent and do not choose any of
their ways.

Proverbs 21:7—The violence of the wicked will
sweep them away, because they refuse to do
what is just.

Approximately four hundred years after Moses imparted the
word of God to the nation of Israel, imploring them to be just
with each other and look to every person's welfare, civil unrest
tore the nation into two parts—the Northern Kingdom,
consisting of ten tribes, and the Southern Kingdom, with the
remaining two tribes of Judah and Benjamin. Both kingdoms
were exemplified by a national character contrary to what Moses
had taught God's people.

Consequently, according to the biblical record, many
prophets were sent to these two kingdoms to warn the people that
God was not pleased when His statutes and principles are not
followed. The writings of these prophets, arising during the many

decades of national decline for the Northern Kingdom of Israel and its sister kingdom to the south, Judah, are testament to how God feels about nations that do not care for the poor, stranger, widowed, orphaned and ill:

> Isaiah 3:15—What do you mean by crushing my people, by grinding the face of the poor?

> Isaiah 5:20–21—Ah, you who call evil good and good evil, who put darkness for light and light for darkness, who put bitter for sweet and sweet for bitter! Ah, you who are wise in your own eyes, and shrewd in your own sight!

> Isaiah 10:1–2—Ah, you who make iniquitous decrees, who write oppressive statutes, to turn aside the needy from justice and to rob the poor of my people of their right, that widows may be your spoil, and that you may make the orphans your prey!

> Isaiah 11:3–4—He shall not judge by what his eyes see, or decide by what his ears hear; but with righteousness he shall judge the poor, and decide with equity for the meek of the earth.

> Isaiah 25:4–5—For you have been a refuge to the poor, a refuge to the needy in their distress, a shelter from the rainstorm and a shade from the heat. When the blast of the ruthless was like a winter rainstorm, the noise of aliens like heat in a dry place, you subdued the heat with the shade of clouds; the song of the ruthless was stilled.

Isaiah 35:3—Strengthen the weak hands, and
make firm the feeble knees.

Isaiah 58:6–7—Is not this the fast that I choose: to
loose the bonds of injustice, to undo the
thongs of the yoke, to let the oppressed go
free, and to break every yoke? Is it not to share
your bread with the hungry, and bring the
homeless poor into your house; when you see
the naked, to cover them, and not to hide
yourself from your own kin?

Jeremiah 7:5–6—For if you truly amend your
ways and your doings, if you truly act justly
one with another, if you do not oppress the
alien, the orphan, and the widow, or shed
innocent blood in this place, neither walk after
other gods to your hurt:

Ezekiel 34:2–4—Ah, you shepherds of Israel who
have been feeding yourselves! Should not
shepherds feed the sheep? You eat the fat, you
clothe yourselves with the wool, you slaughter
the fatlings; but you do not feed the sheep. You
have not strengthened the weak, you have not
healed the sick, you have not bound up the
injured, you have not brought back the
strayed, you have not sought the lost, but with
force and harshness you have ruled them.

Ezekiel 45:9—Enough, O princes of Israel! Put
away violence and oppression and do what is
just and right. Cease your evictions of my
people.

Hosea 12:6—Hold fast to love and justice.

Amos 5:24—But let justice roll down like waters,
and righteousness like an ever-flowing stream.

Micah 6:8—O mortal, what is good; and what
does the Lord require of you but to do justice,
and to love kindness, and to walk humbly with
your God?

Zechariah 7:9–10—Render true judgments, show
kindness and mercy to one another; do not
oppress the widow, the orphan, the alien, or
the poor; and do not devise evil in your hearts
against one another.

Zechariah 8:16–17—These are the things that
you shall do: Speak the truth to one another,
render in your gates judgments that are true
and make for peace, do not devise evil in your
hearts against one another, and love no false
oath.

Jesus, who for Christians is the central figure of the Bible,
anticipated by the Old Testament and coming to life in the New
Testament, went about doing good during His earthly ministry.
He emphasized through His miracles how to serve the sick and
care for the poor who were without food and drink. Whether or
not you believe Jesus was a doer of miracles is not as relevant for
understanding the meaning of the Bible as is the historical
understanding that the people of His time believed He was a
miracle worker.

During His lifetime, Jesus was accused of using the power of
Satan (the devil) to perform His miracles. This was intended as a

damning denial of the goodness of Jesus of Nazareth, but it had the paradoxical effect of confirming that even His enemies conceded that these miracles did occur. And Jesus's friends who wrote the gospel stories about His life included in their writings references to these damning charges from their opponents, something they would not have done lightly given the serious nature of the charge of devilry. Obviously, therefore, both friends and foes accepted as fact that the miracles occurred.

When Jesus invoked whatever were these special talents of His, they were apparently used principally to heal people from injury and illness. Care of the sick and injured was the signature gift of the man known as Jesus of Nazareth. Generations of Christians, up to the recent times in the United States when the for-profit business model of the medical-industrial complex displaced the value of altruistic caring for the sick with avarice, have followed the example of Jesus of Nazareth and provided for the care and nurture of the sick and injured.

Americans have generally induced those elected to positions of governance to spend generously in giving the gift of health care to themselves and their fellow Americans. Here are some of the biblical passages that have inspired these gifts:

> Matthew 9:35—Then Jesus went about all the
> cities and villages, teaching in their syna-
> gogues, and proclaiming the good news of the
> kingdom, and curing every disease and every
> sickness.

> Matthew 11:28–30—Come to me, all you that are
> weary and are carrying heavy burdens, and I
> will give you rest. Take my yoke upon you, and
> learn from me; for I am gentle and humble in
> heart, and you will find rest for your souls. For
> my yoke is easy, and my burden is light.

Matthew 15:30—Great crowds came to him,
   bringing with them the lame, the maimed, the
   blind, the mute, and many others. They put
   them at his feet, and he cured them.

Jesus finished His public teaching just prior to His
   Crucifixion with a parable explicitly
   addressed, unusual for Him, not to individual
   people but to nations:

Matthew 25:31–46—When the Son of Man
   comes in his glory, and all the angels with him,
   then he will sit on the throne of his glory. All
   the nations will be gathered before him, and
   he will separate people one from another as a
   shepherd separates the sheep from the goats,
   and he will put the sheep at his right hand and
   the goats at the left. Then the king will say to
   those at his right hand, "Come, you that are
   blessed by my Father, inherit the kingdom
   prepared for you from the foundation of the
   world; for I was hungry and you gave me food,
   I was thirsty and you gave me something to
   drink, I was a stranger and you welcomed me,
   I was naked and you gave me clothing, I was
   sick and you took care of me, I was in prison
   and you visited me." Then the righteous will
   answer him, "Lord, when was it that we saw
   you hungry and gave you food, or thirsty and
   gave you something to drink? And when was it
   that we saw you a stranger and welcomed you,
   or naked and gave you clothing? And when
   was it that we saw you sick or in prison and
   visited you?" And the king will answer them,

"Truly I tell you, just as you did it to one of
the least of these who are members of my
family, you did it to me." Then he will say to
those at his left hand, "You that are accursed,
depart from me into the eternal fire prepared
for the devil and his angels; for I was hungry
and you gave me no food, I was thirsty and
you gave me nothing to drink, I was a stranger
and you did not welcome me, naked and you
did not give me clothing, sick and in prison
and you did not visit me." Then they also will
answer, "Lord, when was it that we saw you
hungry or thirsty or a stranger or naked or
sick or in prison, and did not take care of
you?" Then he will answer them, "Truly I tell
you, just as you did not do it to one of the least
of these, you did not do it to me." And these
will go away into eternal punishment, but the
righteous into eternal life.

The parable of the sheep and the goats, from which the
above is taken, is a declarative statement about what is meant by
the constitutional assertion that "we the people" should be about
perfecting union, establishing justice, ensuring domestic tranquility, providing for the common defense, promoting the general
welfare, and securing the blessings of liberty. We are not a free
people if among us are those who are hungry, thirsty, isolated,
unclothed (or unhoused), imprisoned, sick, or injured (and
untreated). Without meeting the basic needs of all, we can have
no union, justice, or tranquility.

We cannot defend a society characterized by disunion, injustice, and disrupted harmony. In such a society, general welfare is
unattainable and the blessings of liberty are a mere figment of
the imagination. Our collective failure to achieve a consistent

offering of food, drink, and clothing (or housing) to those without, is, by itself, reprehensible. But we have particularly failed when it comes to visiting those in prison, taking care of those who are sick, or welcoming those who are strangers among us.

Original American conservatism, reliant as it is upon biblical wisdom, would remind us today that we are failing to strengthen the weak, heal the sick, bind up the injured, bring back those who have strayed, and seek the lost but instead are ruling with force and harshness. Hands are hanging down, and knees are feeble, and we don't care. We cannot expect the blessings of peace and protection if we are unwilling to accept our mandated national responsibilities as articulated by Jesus of Nazareth.

"For the hurt of my poor people I am hurt, I mourn, and dismay has taken hold of me. Is there no balm in Gilead? Is there no physician there? Why then has the health of my poor people not been restored?" (Jeremiah 8:20–22). This time of agony will end for us when we give the gift of health care to ourselves, all of us, all the time. We can choose to restore the health of our people.

13

MAXIMUM EFFORT

O n Thursday, June 24, 2021, my daughter Hillary and I left my house in Salt Lake City early in the morning to drive to Big Mountain, which is located east past Emigration Canyon at the top of East Canyon. As we wound up the switchback road in East Canyon, it was raining lightly. The forecast on the evening news the night before had predicted very light rain in the morning and cool temperatures, making for what we hoped was a perfect day of hiking.

Having left my Jeep at the parking lot where the Great Western Trail intersects the Mormon Pioneer Trail at the top of East Canyon, we returned home in time to recruit my wife to drive us the full five-and-a-half-mile length of the paved road in City Creek Canyon and drop us off at the Rotary Park picnic pavilion.

Along the way, we passed the City Creek Canyon water-treatment plant just more than three miles up from the gate to the canyon. City Creek was the first water source used by Brigham Young and the first company of Latter-day Saint pioneers in the nineteenth century. About twenty years after Brigham Young first hand-dipped water for domestic use, City Creek water was distributed by piping for fire protection and culinary supply. Chlorine was added to this piped water supply in 1917. The water-treatment facilities were first constructed in 1953 and were Utah's first municipally owned operation of their kind.

The City Creek watershed consists of 19.2 square miles of canyon upstream from the treatment plant. Rainfall filters through the canyon ecosystem, which has been designated as a protected watershed and nature preserve. The perennial flow of City Creek Canyon yields high-quality water, which I drink myself, living as I do not far from this watershed, which I view as a gift from God to His children.

Like the children of Israel when they took up residence in the land of Canaan, Utahns today depend on rainfall for our livelihood and the stability of our society. Said God to the Israelites:

> "If you follow my statutes and keep my
>   commandments and observe them faithfully, I
>   will give you your rains in their season, and
>   the land shall yield its produce, and the trees
>   of the field shall yield their fruit. Your
>   threshing shall overtake the vintage, and the
>   vintage shall overtake the sowing; you shall eat
>   your bread to the full, and live securely in your
>   land. And I will grant peace in the land, and
>   you shall lie down, and no one shall make you
>   afraid." (Leviticus 26:3–6)

After arriving at the picnic pavilion two miles upstream from the treatment plant, we began our fifteen-mile hike uphill to the top of City Creek Canyon with reverence for what we were about to see and experience. This hike was the reverse of the adventure we had undertaken four years before when I mistakenly led Hillary and her sister Margaret and Margaret's then-boyfriend (now husband) Forrest Strech into the canyon north of City Creek Canyon, where we eventually had to be rescued by helicopter.

By starting in City Creek Canyon, I reasoned that we could not get lost. Even if the trail became difficult to follow, as long as we walked uphill, we would eventually intersect the Great Western Trail. And if we then turned right, we could not fail to find our ride waiting for us where we could see the Salt Lake Valley out in the distance to the west of Big Mountain.

The rain began to fall hard as we left the Rotary Park picnic grounds and headed up the well-marked trail. Within a couple of hundred yards, our feet were soaked, but we trod on, passing the trail ascending two miles to Smugglers Gap, which is between City Creek Canyon and the canyon to the south, Red Butte Canyon. I had hiked that trail years before when my son Andrew and I looped around and over Little Black Mountain on the day City Creek Canyon had been threatened by wildfire. I had also been up the City Creek Canyon trail past the turnoff to Smugglers Gap a couple of years before Hillary and I undertook our hike. But back then I had hiked in the fall when the creek in the upper canyon itself was mostly dry.

Though snowfall totals in the Wasatch Mountains had been low the winter before our hike, Hillary and I found ourselves crossing and recrossing City Creek with a substantial stream flowing, perhaps augmented by the rainfall soaking us through. Our progress was steady for about three miles, and the uphill gradient was not particularly steep.

We were surrounded by late-spring greenery made intense by the fresh precipitation. It was a vibrant, energizing color that drew us uphill through the rain and on into an aspen grove. Dots of color from multivarious wildflowers raised my spirits still higher. I gave the rainfall no heed and slopped on uphill. I did transfer my wallet, already soaking wet, from my pocket to a watertight compartment in Hillary's pack. She was already carrying the lion's share of the water and calorie supplies, which consisted of protein bars, protein drinks, and sport beans.

There is a kind of plateau at the top of City Creek Canyon called the Meadows between Lookout Mountain to the south and Grandview Mountain to the north. The mile before reaching that plateau is steeper on the trail, which is still well-marked there. This steeper section of trail above the aspen grove was as far as I had hiked the fall two years before. It was in this section of trail that we began finding trees fallen and splayed like so many matchsticks, most still producing the green leaves of spring while prone. I presumed that these fallen trees had been victimized by the hurricane-force winds that had accompanied a low-pressure weather system from the east in early September 2020.

Beginning just before we arrived at the Meadow and continuing across its two-mile scope, we had to negotiate our way around, over, or under many fallen trees that blocked the trail. I found myself having to remove my small trail pack to get under a tree trunk, and even then I had difficulty with crawling and bending. Trying to scramble over a tree was even more difficult. At my age, I was no longer spry. Where possible, I took a route around a fallen tree.

When we emerged from the steeper trail out onto the Meadows, there were fewer fallen trees. The view toward the top of the canyon was expansive, with the Meadows cradled between Lookout and Grandview mountains. The rain lightened, and with the clouds breaking up, the verdant meadow foliage took on the emerald sheen of virescence. We could see the rise toward the very eastern rim of the canyon off in the distance. I expected to very soon find the location where I had misled my small hiking group four years before.

Just then, the trail became less well marked, more difficult to relocate if a tree detour was needed, and we became less clear about our path forward. For a time, we followed a dry creek bed, always going uphill, as planned. However, the thickened foliage around the creek bed and rocky creek bottom itself became increasingly difficult to navigate.

Then we thought we had a trail to follow, which angled off to the north toward the lower slopes of Grandview Mountain. But as that path became steeper, it petered out. We picked our way slowly through the underbrush back toward the canyon bottom. Bushwhacking is an exhausting way to hike. The nettles stung my legs with every step. Missteps onto rocks or into burrows were common because I couldn't see the ground. And as we were trying to ascend the canyon, every step was uphill anyway. I began to feel the shakiness that for me is always a preamble to muscle cramping. And just then we found ourselves cornered between a steep mountainside and a dense thicket of brush and trees around the creek bed.

I asked for a protein bar and chewed slowly, then washed it down with water, still icy cold in the coolness of the day. Hillary was a willing companion, game to try whatever looked feasible for our next foray forward. So, because I didn't think I could bushwhack my way through the creek bed, I chose to scramble up the steep mountainside by pulling myself up and forward, grasping whatever scrub plants seemed strong enough to bear my weight. It was, for me, a maximal effort, which I continued to give until we climbed high enough to see our way around the thicket beneath us.

We traveled sideways around the slope of the hill until we alighted in a clearing that stood before another hill that divided the canyon in two. Here I again needed hydration, nourishment, and rest. Hillary was still willing to push onward even though we had not seen a trail for a couple of miles.

I suggested we climb the hill, gain the view from the top, and make a better-informed decision about the way forward. The hillside was steep but less so than the scrub-plant-grasping maximal effort. Hillary had no trouble negotiating it and arrived at the top well before I did. Once I joined her, she pointed out a herd of twenty-five elk grazing a half mile away toward the north on the slopes of Grandview Mountain. Just as I spotted them, they broke into a run and disappeared behind a veil of trees.

I looked toward the southeast and saw the sloped open area I knew instantly to be the place where I had misled my hiking group four years before. That spot was down below us in altitude and across the upper portion of the Meadow, which was now narrowing. Above it there was what appeared to be dense forest. We chose to hike along the north side of the Meadow toward the forest while losing as little altitude as possible, with the theory that every step of descent would require a compensatory two steps of ascent to regain lost elevation.

Finally, we edged our way into the forest and found it relatively free of brush. Using the tree trunks for leverage, I climbed the final two hundred yards of City Creek Canyon and stepped out onto its east rim, looking out over the back side of the Wasatch Front—a panoramic eastward view. The Great Western Trail was before me on the rim.

We turned right, as had been the plan, and lit out for the slopes of Big Mountain about seven miles away. This was the trail we had taken in reverse four years ago, and we recognized its features, sights, and scenes. We saw the place where we had skirted a snowbank. Now, four years later, after a dismally low snowfall during winter, the spot was bone dry. We walked past the sign that marked the limit of the City Creek Canyon watershed and warned hikers about restrictions protecting the water supply for Salt Lake City.

We edged around the circumference of a steep-sided bowl that formed the upper portion of a branch of East Canyon, tucked behind and to the east of Emigration Canyon. There, the trail treacherously faded away for a couple of steps in three places, requiring me to gingerly search for semisolid footing and somewhere to surge forward. Ultimately, the trail joined with a Jeep road, along which signs were posted announcing that the downhill slope to the east was part of a private resort preserve and not to be trespassed.

After several miles, the Great Western Trail separates from the Jeep road and heads uphill, beginning the ascent that eventually peaks below the summit of Big Mountain. Hillary and I reached this renewed uphill trek midafternoon. Suddenly, the sun was blotted out by dark clouds, and thunder started rolling and echoing, gaining volume with each volley. As we climbed, the clouds reached down from the sky and covered the trail, embracing us and obscuring our view. The wind picked up, the temperature fell, and I could smell the moisture condensing for a few minutes before the rain started.

Hillary, in particular, was freezing, but she soldiered on. Because we had been there before, we knew we were closing in on our objective. She would soon warm herself with a heated seat in the Jeep. I was completely spent. Fifteen miles over seven hours, mostly uphill, and I had nothing left to give to the trail. We were cold and wet, but we did not need a helicopter to save me from exhaustion. The last mile of the trail was downhill. We emerged from the cloud, dipped below the mountain ridge and out of the wind, then switchbacked down to highway level. We'd made it.

My nation has a heavy political lift ahead. Seventy-five years ago, when we were gifting to the people of Europe the Marshall Plan and writing a democratic constitution for the citizens of Japan, we should have done ourselves the favor of eliminating the tax credits for employer-based health benefits. Like the exhausted people of Great Britain in the aftermath of WWII, we should have organized public funding for health care—not coverage—for every American. The British opted for the National Health Service, a truly socialized health system. We would have chosen differently had we been as kind to ourselves as we were to our allies and former enemies. Instead, we allowed the for-profit, private health-insurance business model—the most useless, avaricious, health-financing scheme ever invented—to take root in America just as the power of clinical medicine became manifest.

Like a cancer, health insurers grew from community-rated, nonprofit payers for care regulated by state governments to massive investor-owned, windfall-profiteering, corporate cash cows feeding at the national public trough and writing public law and appropriations to please themselves. Every effort my nation has made since then to do something about the growing metastasis of for-profit health insurance has been to the benefit of the medical-industrial complex because they use corporate welfare to lock down legislation, appropriations, and all government processes to generate more corporate welfare.

Excising this seventy-five-year-old malignancy from the body politic of the United States of America will require maximum effort, like scrambling from bush to bush up the highest slopes of City Creek Canyon in the rain. Just like I missed the trail four years ago and failed to complete my intended trek, the Greatest Generation came home from WWII and failed to see the danger in an arcane tax policy that favored health insurance as an employment benefit.

Baby Boomers like me grew up experiencing a widening array of clinical victories and allowed health-insurance branding to make us believe that what we needed was coverage. But subsequent generations, millennials and GenXers, now know better. Jobs haven't been as plentiful for them, and when those jobs are available, they are not as rich in health benefits. Health benefits, when offered, are now hollowed-out, empty promises. Corporate for-profit hospitals and practices would rather make a sale than care for us; there is both too much medical intervention and not enough for the good of our patients, who are frequently injured while supposedly receiving care. And we Americans fund all of this through taxation. We pay for care we never receive.

Ever since John McCain gave a thumbs-down to the so-called "skinny" repeal of the Affordable Care Act about four years ago, my former political party, the Republicans, has not wanted to talk about healthcare policy. The "skinny" repeal was short for "repeal but don't replace," referring to the Affordable Care Act. At the time he voted no on the repeal, John McCain clearly articulated how empty the promises of his Republican colleagues were.

McCain summed up the political challenge of health-system reform in a nutshell. Health insurance is a mess despite Obamacare, or perhaps because of it. Changing healthcare business as usual requires a consensus. While Republicans clearly have nothing useful to say about health-system reform, it is not better for Democrats to talk about it but do nothing when in office.

Governing elites have been ignoring the care needed for the sick and injured to enrich themselves for at least three thousand years. The Old Testament prophet Ezekiel, who ministered to captured Israel as they labored on the giant public-works projects of Babylon, spoke to the failings of the governing elite in the kingdom of Judah leading to the fall of Jerusalem. He said, "You have not strengthened the weak, you have not healed the sick, you have not bound up the injured, you have not brought back the strayed, you have not sought the lost, but with force and harshness you have ruled" us (Ezekiel 34:4). A couple of decades before the Babylonian burning of Jerusalem, Ezekiel's senior prophet associate, Jeremiah, offered that indictment of the cruelty of Judean rule: "For the hurt of my poor people I am hurt, I mourn, and dismay has taken hold of me. Is there no balm in Gilead? Is there no physician there? Why then has the health of my poor people not been restored?" (Jeremiah 8:20–22).

Like Jeremiah, I hurt for the hurt of my people. With Ezekiel, I call out the force and harshness of business as usual in American health care. For more than seventy-five years, the American people have had their health care increasingly hijacked by profiteering businesses. To be sure, healthcare services have improved during that same period of time, but that is because American taxpayers have had the goodness and altruism to fund basic laboratory research, clinical science, medical and nursing education, and the building of health structures in every corner of the country. We Americans have made our clinical care better despite the hijacking by for-profit healthcare businesses. There *is* a balm in Gilead and a physician or nurse who knows how to apply it.

But we as a society are not applying the balm of Gilead. I believe the stark political divisions in our country now trending toward violence have health-system failure as a principal cause. As mentioned—and I am repeating it here to make sure it is clearly understood—it was poor health and a consequently rising death rate among white, middle-aged, non-college-educated voters, many living in rural areas, that brought Donald Trump the relatively few crossover votes he needed to win the presidential election in 2016. Trump's surprise victory that year came at the same time life expectancy dropped for the United States for the first time in my lifetime due exclusively to a half million excess deaths among white Americans under age sixty-five while death rates among black Americans and Hispanics were improving.

Several observers, among them Nobel Laureate Angus Deaton, have noted that the declining mortality figures among white non-college-educated Americans can be attributed to drug and alcohol overdoses, which almost quadrupled; suicides, which increased by 60 percent; and deaths from chronic liver disease and cirrhosis, which rose by a third. Thus, these deaths have been labeled deaths of despair. As Jeff Goldsmith sums it up:

"In plainer words, white Americans in mid-life are basically killing themselves, either directly or with destructive personal habits, and in sufficient numbers to affect overall life expectancy in the country. It is not challenging to link the despair of older voters to de-industrialization and the economic hammering many Americans took in the 2008 recession, and thus to Trump's surprise victory."[1]

If we are to counter the trend toward the violence of those claiming to have our best interests at heart and heal our nation, we must address the underlying decay causing increased morbidity and mortality among us. At least twice in the past—in 1861 and 1933, when America was at its most divisive, these lowest points caused respectively by secession and depression, subsequent armed conflict unified the nation's resolve to save itself. And after the travail of battle leading to victory, in each case costing hundreds of thousands of American lives, the nation engaged in an outpouring of generosity for the vanquished enemy and reaffirmation of the virtues of constitutional governance at home, followed by a time of peace and prosperity. It is worth remembering what Abraham Lincoln said in the aftermath of the Civil War:

"With malice toward none; with charity for all; with firmness in the right, as God gives us to see the right, let us strive on to finish the work we are in; to bind up the nation's wounds; to care for him who shall have borne the battle, and for his widow, and his orphan—to do all which may achieve and cherish a just, and a lasting peace, among ourselves, and with all nations."[2]

Reconstruction after the Civil War and the Marshall Plan after WWII were not preordained policies. In fact, over the world history of armed conflict, it is the rare victor who has made sacrifices to help heal the wounds of war suffered by a defeated people.

We Americans are again at a defining moment in our history. We are again at a low in governance. We are divided by malice and mischief. We have fought in the Middle East for twenty years. Hundreds of thousands of us have died unexpectedly during the past year.

We need to make a down payment of goodness and charity sufficient to, as Lincoln put it, "bind up the nation's wounds" and "do all which may achieve and cherish a just, and a lasting peace, among ourselves, and with all nations." We need reconstruction and a Marshall Plan for ourselves, the exhausted and maimed society that has survived our self-inflicted near destruction.

What we need is a way to tangibly and reliably care for ourselves. We need to put hands on each other and reach out to heal.

Again, let me repeat: No matter which faction or tribe any one of us might adhere to, no matter how unfairly treated we each perceive ourselves individually to be, no matter how unloved or unloving we might be, we can offer the balm of Gilead to one another. We can choose to wrest the ownership of health care away from the medical-industrial complex and restore it to its original purpose—to act with charity in every American life. We need no new appropriations; we have long since taxed ourselves heavily for health care. The public revenue streams already exist. We must simply decide, in paraphrase of President Truman, that a "principal concern of the people of the United States is the creation of conditions of enduring" health.

To do this, we must remove the for-profit motive from health-care delivery. For-profit businesses would rather make a sale than care for a patient, so they invent new ways to induce the purchase of narcotics and walk away from the opiate addiction epidemic that follows. For-profit businesses would rather make blockbuster profits by extending patent rights by fiddling with already-known pharmaceuticals, so we have infinite variations of stomach-acid-reducing drugs and no new antibiotics. For-profit businesses would rather charge the price, no matter how high, that optimizes their profits than see to it that every patient who needs a medication can afford it. And, not surprisingly, deaths due to very treatable conditions like diabetes and hypertension happen all too often.

For-profit businesses know which parts of the hospital are most lucrative, so intensive care is preferred over prevention and primary care. Caring for patients is principally a labor of skilled professionals, but labor costs undermine the highest profits, so for-profit healthcare businesses do everything they can to reduce their labor costs without regard to patient safety. The consequence is at least 250,000 premature deaths per year due to preventable injury of hospitalized patients.

America's de facto health-financing business scheme, health insurance driven by profits, was made financially solvent seventy-five years ago only by granting the industry a then-unprecedented massive federal tax credit, valued today at around $500 billion per year. Despite that massive annual subsidy, the health-insurance industry has, over the years, persuaded Congress to allow them to cherry-pick the healthy while the taxpayers shoulder the financial responsibility for the care of the elderly, the poor, children, veterans, and Obamacare health plans. Nonetheless, despite paying the world's highest taxes for health care, Americans are by the tens of millions uninsured and underinsured, leading to fifty thousand deaths per year and hundreds of thousands of personal and family bankruptcies. For the hurt of my people, I am hurt.

These are facts. Costs in the United States for health care are ridiculously high. No other first-world nation puts up with the costs, poor quality, and inefficiency that is rampant in American healthcare business as usual. No other first-world nation allows diabetics to go without insulin because of cost. Ambulance services don't bankrupt patients in any first-world nation other than the United States. Americans pay the world's highest taxes for health care but are the least likely in the first world to survive conditions treatable by known clinical science. Better, simpler, and therefore cheaper health-system reform, successfully implemented in many other first-world countries and widely studied economically in the United States, is a superior patient-care option for healthcare delivery at a lower price because it is more efficient and fosters better quality care.

The question is no longer whether the United States health-care system is underperforming. It is. Nor does anyone doubt that health care in the United States is far too expensive. That is undisputedly true. Nor is there a serious debate about whether real, sustainable health-system reform would address the cost problems of health care in the United States. The real question before every American is how we can finally develop the political will to do the reform we need when the trillions of healthcare dollars we generously spend through taxation, employer benefits, and personal out-of-pocket costs are being used against us to defend the sick status quo in American health care. With Ezekiel, the Old Testament prophet, we say to our political leaders and the owners and operators of the medical-industrial complex, "You have not strengthened the weak, you have not healed the sick, you have not bound up the injured, you have not brought back the strayed, you have not sought the lost, but with force and harshness you have ruled" us (Ezekiel 34:4).

There is no roadmap for reforming the massive American health system. No other social movement in the history of our country has faced the likes of the wealth and power of the American medical-industrial complex, so entrenched as it is in the business community at large and so interwoven into the fabric of our two major political parties.

WHAT YOU CAN DO

Here are my personal priorities for furthering the movement toward a sustainable American health policy:

1. Remember what John McCain said.

At a minimum, I never support a candidate for public office who does not reiterate what John McCain said: "Our health care insurance system is a mess. We all know it, those who support Obamacare and those who oppose it. Something has to be done." And then a candidate, if she wants my support, must go on to openly and repeatedly support state-based health-system reform. I helped Kathy Allen, a Utah Democrat, during her special election race for Congress in 2018, but I later regretted it because she failed the state-based test. I spoke with both Shireen Ghorbani and Kael Weston, both Democrats running for Congress to unseat Chris Stewart during their campaigns, and eventually donated to Mr. Weston when he placed an endorsement of state-based reform on his campaign website. I always vote, and if I find no candidate in a race upon whom I can rely for support of real, sustainable health-system reform, I vote to un-elect the incumbent because an incumbent has already failed. I do not ever consider party affiliation when voting; my only consideration is tangible evidence of support for health reform characterized by regionally cooperative, high-quality, privately delivered health care guaranteed by unified, simplified public health-system financing.

2. Lobby for the federal superwaiver legislation needed to free states to take on comprehensive health-system reform.

Ro Khanna (D-CA) has introduced this legislation into the current session of Congress. When he did so in the previous Congress, the *New York Times* reported: "Federal rules can make it difficult for states to create single payer systems. . . . The Khanna legislation . . . envisions a waiver that would allow states to take over the Medicare money that flows their way and combine it with funding for Medicaid, the Affordable Care Act market-places, the Tricare program that covers military families and funds for veterans' health care. A state would need to submit a plan for how it would use those funds to cover at least 95% of its population within five years, then cover the remaining uninsured within a decade."[1] That sounds like a plan that would attract Republicans. I have personally discussed this legislation with Blake Moore and John Curtis, Republican members of the United States House of Representatives from Utah, and with staff in the offices of Senator Mitt Romney and Senator Mike Lee. Every Utahn should join me in this lobbying effort. We need a Utah Member of Congress to endorse this legislation during the current Congress.

3. Put real, sustainable health-system reform on the ballot.

I will do what I can to have Utah join the twenty-one other states that have organized movements toward better, simpler, and therefore cheaper health-system reform by ballot initiative. More details about this are available in my book, *The Purple World: Healing the Harm in American Health Care*. I am currently trying to organize an economic study of the effect such reform will have in Utah, including answering significant questions such as the following: How much tax money (federal, state, local) is already spent on health care where I live? How much money could be saved by simplifying healthcare administration through reform that unifies and simplifies health-system payments? How much money could be saved by improving the quality of health care in my local hospitals? You can tangibly assist me with this process by pledging to donate to defray the costs of the study.

4. Sustainable health-system reform is the sentinel domestic issue of our time, not merely a progressive plank.

I will not be distracted from health-system reform by other issues or causes, no matter how worthy. Yes, the climate is under threat, but we are losing at least 250,000 lives per year now because of abysmal health-system performance. Of course, Black Lives Matter, but every oppressed and alienated American will be blessed by hands-on care if, and only if, our health system is sustainably improved. Whether one is pro-life or pro-choice, better health care for every woman will improve her health and that of every child she chooses to bring into the world and will make less likely the occurrence of abortion. Every aspect of American life will be substantially improved by real health-system reform. America is and will be only as great as the care it provides to the sick and injured. Ask Ezekiel and Jeremiah.

5. Remember the Johnstown flood.

Act on the assumption that the status quo in health care cannot long continue because the flood of waste and lost lives is unsustainable. For perspective, remember the Johnstown, Pennsylvania, flood of 1889. To sum up what we already discussed, on May 31 of that year, a dam failed fourteen miles upstream from Johnstown, an industrial city in western Pennsylvania of about thirty thousand people. A sixty-foot wall of water crashed into the town and in ten minutes killed nearly three thousand people and caused $20 billion in damage (in 2020 dollars). I never forget that twice each week, business as usual in American health care kills as many Americans as died in the Johnstown flood, and three times each month, poor-quality care and inefficiency in health-care delivery wastes as much money as was lost through damage in the Johnstown flood. The stupid way we fund health care harms our businesses, governments, and families. It locks people into jobs, reduces productivity, and keeps them from having families and owning homes. As big as is the American economy, it will eventually fall apart from the deluge of harm caused by American health care as it currently is. The cracks in the economy caused by massive health-system waste are already hard to hide and will widen and deepen in the coming few years. American for-profit health insurance as a business model adds nothing of value to the American way of life, and it will be thrown on the trash heap of history. American healthcare business as usual is not sustainable.

6. Seek to create a Harris Wofford moment.

Thirty years ago, when I first became acquainted with the strength of the published health-policy literature that supports improved quality care guaranteed by unified and simplified health care, I was persuaded by political events in Pennsylvania that the nation was preparing to elect leadership that would bring about the needed health-system changes. In 1991, then Democratic governor of Pennsylvania, Robert Casey, announced the appointment of Harris Wofford to fill a vacated United States Senate seat and run in a special election to finish the term.

Wofford, despite serving at the time as Pennsylvania Labor and Industry secretary, was an unknown and a first-time candidate. He had served on the staff of John F. Kennedy's presidential campaign and enjoyed some success in bringing African-American voters to support the Democratic ticket for the first time. But he was a novice running against a veteran politician who had the backing of President George H. W. Bush.

Wofford was given no chance of winning the special election. The first poll taken in the very short campaign had him down by forty-seven points. Wofford gamely took on the domestic policies of the first Bush administration and stumbled on a line that repeatedly gave him the applause he craved: "The Constitution says that if you are charged with a crime, you have a right to a lawyer. But it's even more fundamental that if you're sick, you should have the right to a doctor."[2] Wofford rode that line and the Pennsylvania public's craving for healthcare security to a 55 to 45 percent win, a totally unexpected political victory that sent shock waves through the nation.

For the first time, it appeared the American public had an appetite for health-system reform. Wofford later said, "Until I had that victory, people weren't seeing [health care] as the big issue. And [Bill] Clinton called me the day after I was elected . . . [and] he hadn't settled on health care as a big campaign issue." [3]

In 1991, when Wofford came out of nowhere to win the special election, erasing a forty-point polling deficit, and changed the national political conversation, it seemed to me that healthcare reform could be a winning political strategy and that one well-placed United States Senate race could refocus the entire nation's political discourse. The two presidents who succeeded Mr. Clinton, George W. Bush and Barack Obama, both featured health reform prominently in their initial campaigns. Bush, contrary to typical Republican dogma, favored expanding Medicare to provide a medication benefit, and Obama spoke to increasing "coverage." Even Trump nodded to the necessity of supporting public financing of health care with his against-the-Republican-grain promise to not "'reform" Medicare by narrowing its benefits even while promising to repeal Obamacare.

Politicians from both major parties are vulnerable to healthcare insurgencies because both parties pander to the profiteering of the medical-industrial complex. Therefore, I will take every opportunity I can to speak out about state-based, better, simpler, cheaper health-system reform. I will use every medium available. I maintain social media accounts (Facebook—Dr Joe Jarvis; Twitter—@DrJoeQJarvis) to connect with the thousands of Americans nationwide who are already in this effort. I will start and maintain a political action committee built to support candidates who will change American health care and state ballot initiatives that will bring that change home to all Americans. I will be a part of the next Harris Wofford moment in American politics.

I hope you all will be there to join me when that moment comes.

NOTES

2. AVARICE VERSUS ALTRUISM

1. Dana Miller Ervin, "Here's Why Insulin Costs So Much in the U.S.," WFAE, February 23, 2021.
2. Ervin.

3. STATE-BASED HEALTH REFORM: WHAT CONSERVATIVES BELIEVE

1. Theodore Roosevelt, https://www.theodorerooseveltcenter.org/Research/Digital-Library/Record?libID=o279386. Theodore Roosevelt Digital Library. Dickinson State University.
2. Barry M. Goldwater, as quoted in Dick Armey and Matt Kibbe, Give Us Liberty: A Tea Party Manifesto, HarperCollins e-books
3. Barry M. Goldwater, The Conscience of a Conservative, Princeton University Press, 1960.
4. Ibid.
5. Goldwater, *Excerpts From Goldwater Remarks". Remarks in the Congressional Record, www.nytimes.com. September 15, 1981*
6. Ibid.
7. Goldwater, https://www.nytimes.com/1993/06/11/us/goldwater-backs-gay-troops.html
8. Goldwater, The conscience of a majority (ed. Prentice Hall, 1970)
9. Goldwater, The Conscience of a Conservative, Princeton University Press, 1960.
10. Ibid.
11. Theodore Roosevelt, "The New Nationalism," in *The New Nationalism* (New York: The Outlook Company, 1910)
12. Theodore Roosevelt, *(2015). "Theodore Roosevelt on Bravery: Lessons from the Most Courageous Leader of the Twentieth Century", p.78, Skyhorse Publishing, Inc.*

4. RUNNING THROUGH THE POLITICAL ICEBOX

1. Bill Semple, personal communication to the author.
2. Bill Moyers, http://www.pbs.org/moyers/journal/blog/2009/10/bill_moyers_michael_winship_in.html

3. David Graham Phillips, "The Treason of the Senate," 1906.

5. HEALTH CARE: THE SENTINEL DOMESTIC
ISSUE OF OUR TIME

1. John McCain, https://thehill.com/blogs/pundits-blog/healthcare/343694-full-speech-john-mccain-on-key-senate-healthcare-vote/

6. METAPHOR AND HEALING

1. Jeff Goldsmith, "America's Health and the 2016 Election: An Unexpected Connection," The Healthcare Blog, January 4, 2017, https://thehealthcare-blog.com/blog/2017/01/04/americas-health-and-the-2016-election-an-unexpected-connection.
2. See Fritjof Capra, *The Turning Point: Science, Society, and the Rising Culture* (New York: Bantam Books, 1982), 123–63; see also J. T. Edelson, "Metaphor, Medicine, and Medical Education," *Pharos* 47 (Spring, 1984): 16–21; see also Joan M. Boyle and James E. Morriss, "The Philosophical Roots of the Current Medical Crisis," *Metaphilosophy* 12 (1981): 284–301.
3. Colin Turbayne, *The Myth of Metaphor* (Columbia, South Carolina: University of South Carolina Press, 1970), 3, 21, 64, 67.
4. Ibid.
5. Ibid.
6. Ibid.
7. Ibid.
8. Joan M. Boyle and James E. Morriss, "The Philosophical Roots of the Current Medical Crisis," *Metaphilosophy* 12 (1981): 284–301.
9. Susan Sontag, *Illness as Metaphor* (New York: Farrar, Strauss and Giroux, 1977), 5.
10. Franz J. Ingelfinger, "Health: A Matter of Statistics or Feeling," *New England Journal of Medicine* 296 (1977): 448–49.
11. Rene Dubos, *Mirage of Health* (New York: Harper and Row, 1971).
12. Kenneth M. Heilman, Edward Valenstein, *Clinical Neuropsychology* (Oxford: Oxford University Press, 1979), 20.
13. Karl Rogers, "A Theory of Therapy as Developed in the Client-Centered Framework," ed., Ben N. Ard, *Counselling and Psychotherapy: Classics on Theories and Issues* (Palo Alto, California: Science and Behavior Books, Inc., 1966), 49.
14. Harold Bursztajn, Richard Feinbloom, Robert Hamm, and Archie Brodsky, *Medical Choices, Medical Chances: How Patients, Families and Physicians Can Cope with Uncertainty* (New York: Delacourte Press, 1981), 51–52.
15. John Hayes, "Existentialism in Medical Education," *Pharos* 43 (Summer, 1980): 32.
16. Lewis Thomas, *Lives of a Cell* (New York: The Viking Press, 1974), 55–56.
17. John Hayes, "Existentialism in Medical Education," *Pharos* 43 (Summer, 1980): 32.

7. THE METAPHORICAL PHYSICIAN

1. Carl Binger, *The Doctor's Job* (New York: W.W. Norton and Company, Inc., 1945), 14.
2. Carl Binger, *The Two Faces of Medicine* (New York: W. W. Norton and Company, Inc., 1967), 79.
3. Samuel Taylor Coleridge, "Biographia Literaria," in *Major British Writers*, vol. II. ed. Harrison GB (New York: Harcourt, Brace and World, Inc., 1959), 135.
4. Harold Bursztajn, Richard Feinbloom, Robert Hamm, and Archie Brodsky, *Medical Choices, Medical Chances: How Patients, Families and Physicians Can Cope with Uncertainty* (New York: Delacourte Press, 1981), 51–52.
5. Norman Cousins, *Anatomy of an Illness as Perceived by the Patient: Reflections on Healing and Regeneration* (New York: W.W. Norton and Company, Inc., 1979), 48, 149.
6. Kenneth R. Pelletier, *Holistic medicine: From Stress to Optimum Health* (New York: Dell Publishing Company, Inc., 1979), 22, 96–127.
7. Jack J. Leedy, ed., *Poetry therapy: The Use of Poetry in the Treatment of Emotional Disorders* (Philadelphia: JB Lippincott Co., 1969).
8. Kenneth R. Pelletier, *Holistic medicine: From Stress to Optimum Health* (New York: Dell Publishing Company, Inc., 1979), 22, 96–127.
9. Albert Camus, *The Plague*, trans. Stuart Gilbert (New York: Vintage Books, 1972), 179.
10. Norman Cousins, *Anatomy of an Illness as Perceived by the Patient: Reflections on Healing and Regeneration* (New York: W.W. Norton and Company, Inc., 1979), 48, 149.
11. Maia Szalavitz, "I've Covered Drug Policy for Three Decades. Here's Why I'm Looking to Oregon," Guest Essay, *New York Times*, January 26, 2022.

8. THE HOW OF PROGRESS AND CONSERVATIVE HEALTH REFORM

1. Louis Brandeis, *New State Ice Co. v. Liebmann*, 285 U.S. 262, 1932.

9. HARRIS WOFFORD, FORCE, AND HARSHNESS

1. Lara Shore-Sheppard, "Medicaid and CHIP: Filling in the Gap of Children's Health Insurance Coverage," Econofact, January 22, 2018, https://econofact.org/filling-in-the-gap-of-childrens-health-insurance-coverage-medicaid-and-chip.

10. DOWNSTREAM DANGER

1. David McCullough, *The Johnstown Flood* (New York: Simon & Schuster, 1968), 145–47.
2. McCullough, 73–74.
3. McCullough, 224–25.
4. McCullough, 230–31.
5. Dwight Eisenhower, "Remarks at Fourth Annual Republican Women's National Conference."
   American Presidents Project. 6 March 1956.

11. THE BELL TOLLS FOR EVERY AMERICAN

1. Abraham Lincoln, Second Inaugural Address.
2. Edward Delos Churchill, http://history.massgeneral.org/catalog/Detail.aspx?itemId=119&searchFor=churchill
3. Harry S.Truman, https://www.presidency.ucsb.edu/documents/special-message-the-congress-the-marshall-plan
4. See hcao.org.
5. John C. Goodman, *Wall Street Journal*, April 5, 2007.
6. McKinsey and Co, https://www.mckinsey.com/industries/education/our-insights/the-economic-cost-of-the-us-education-gap.

13. MAXIMUM EFFORT

1. Jeff Goldsmith, "America's Health and the 2016 Election: An Unexpected Connection," The Healthcare Blog, January 4, 2017, https://thehealthcare-blog.com/blog/2017/01/04/americas-health-and-the-2016-election-an-unexpected-connection.
2. Abraham Lincoln, Second Inaugural Address

WHAT YOU CAN DO

1. Sarah Kliff, *New York Times*, "What if the Road to Single-Payer Led Through the States?, November 8, 2019.
2. Harris Wofford, https://www.washingtonpost.com/archive/lifestyle/wellness/1991/11/19/the-right-to-see-a-doctor-when-youre-sick/01648b6c-7878-46e4-a8ac-02fb2ecfbe8b/
3. Harris Wofford, https://observer.com/2009/09/a-democratic-casualty-of-clinton-care-thinks-obama-has-it-about-right/.

ABOUT THE AUTHOR

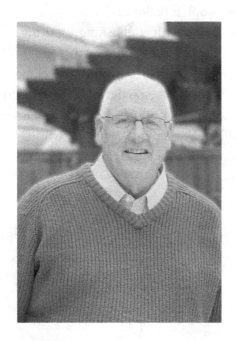

Joseph Q. Jarvis, MD, MSPH has practiced family medicine and organized public health services for over thirty-five years. His spouse of nearly five decades, Annette W. Jarvis, is an internationally recognized business bankruptcy attorney. Together they have five children and nine grandchildren.

Dr. Jarvis is the author of three other books—*The Purple World: Healing the Harm in American Health Care*, *What the Single Eye Sees: Faith, Hope, Charity, and the Pursuit of Discipleship*, and *The Hope of the Promise: Israel in Ancient and Latter Days*. He is the executive producer of *Healing Us*, a documentary film by director Kenny Ballentine about the awful state of business as usual in American health care and how everyday Americans can change it all for the better. Dr. Jarvis is also helping to organize a national political action committee—the American Health Security Project—to support health system reform everywhere across the country and leading a Utah group—Common Sense Health Care for Utah--which intends to make real change in health care delivery in the Beehive State through a ballot initiative.

When not busy with publishing, writing, leading health system reform, or spending time with family, Dr. Jarvis leads tours in Europe and Israel with his travel company, Mo Joe Travel. Dr. Jarvis is also the owner of Principle Print & Media, a company dedicated to producing inspirational and educational content that will make a difference in the world.

Find out more about Dr. Jarvis and sign up for his newsletter at josephqjarvis.com!

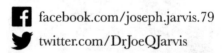

facebook.com/joseph.jarvis.79

twitter.com/DrJoeQJarvis

ALSO BY
JOSEPH Q. JARVIS, MD, MSPH

What the Single Eye Sees: Faith, Hope, Charity, and the Pursuit of Discipleship

Dr. Joseph Q. Jarvis reveals spiritual insights we've never considered, teaches us how to explore what Christ's call to discipleship means, and how following that call deepens our relationship with the Savior.

The Hope of the Promise: Israel in Ancient and Latter Days

Dr. Joseph Q. Jarvis explores the real sites of biblical events, their connection to the gospel, and how we can use them to enrich our faith. Using vivid images and archaeological analysis, he gives context to the stories we were raised with, reminding us that they are a pivotal part of history.

The Purple World: Healing the Harm in American Health Care

Dr. Joseph Q. Jarvis examines how our nation's focus has radically shifted from the disease to the dollar—drastically harming Americans in the process. Instead of simply pointing fingers and wailing about the outrages, Dr. Joseph Q. Jarvis offers a workable solution that can be implemented by each state.

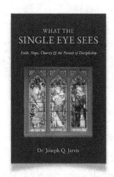

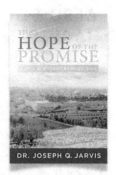

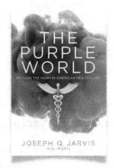

CPSIA information can be obtained
at www.ICGtesting.com
Printed in the USA
BVHW031510140722
642159BV00012BB/815